Cholera in Detroit

ALSO BY RICHARD ADLER
AND FROM MCFARLAND

*Mack, McGraw and the 1913
Baseball Season* (2008)

Cholera in Detroit
A History

RICHARD ADLER

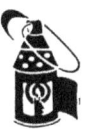

McFarland & Company, Inc., Publishers
Jefferson, North Carolina, and London

LIBRARY OF CONGRESS CATALOGUING-IN-PUBLICATION DATA

Adler, Rich.
    Cholera in Detroit : a history / Richard Adler.
      p.   cm.
    Includes bibliographical references and index.

    ISBN 978-0-7864-7479-0
    softcover : acid free paper ∞

    1. Cholera — Michigan — Detroit — History. 2. Public health — Michigan — Detroit — History. I. Title.
    RC131.M52D483 2013
    614.5'140977434 — dc23   2013026115

BRITISH LIBRARY CATALOGUING DATA ARE AVAILABLE

© 2013 Richard Adler. All rights reserved

No part of this book may be reproduced or transmitted in any form or by any means, electronic or mechanical, including photocopying or recording, or by any information storage and retrieval system, without permission in writing from the publisher.

On the cover: *top* Steamship *Sheldon Thompson*, one of the schooners which transported General Scott and his troops (courtesy Burton Historical Collection, Detroit Public Library); *bottom* reaper timing the next victim (© 2013 clipart.com); *inset* microscopic image of the Vibrio Cholerae organism (courtesy Louisa Howard, Dartmouth College); *background* map of the United States Cholera Route, Epidemic of 1832 (compiled by Ely Mc. Clellan)

Manufactured in the United States of America

McFarland & Company, Inc., Publishers
  Box 611, Jefferson, North Carolina 28640
    www.mcfarlandpub.com

Table of Contents

Acknowledgments   vii
Introduction   1

1. From India to America   9
2. Cholera Crosses the Border   19
3. Cholera Among the Troops   34
4. Detroit, Vintage 1832   42
5. Detroit, Cholera and the Black Hawk War: Events of 1832   54
6. Cholera Returns: 1834   84
7. Between the Cholera "Wars"   101
8. The Epidemic of 1849   115
9. Epidemic of 1854   127
10. Epidemic of 1866: New York, Detroit and Beyond   142
11. The 1870s and Beyond   164
12. Isolation and Identification of the Cholera Bacillus   174
13. Aftermath   191

Chapter Notes   199
Bibliography   213
Index   217

Acknowledgments

I would like to acknowledge the help and support of a number of persons. My wife of course, who proofread some of the material, and who helped remove our two cats which insisted the keyboard of my laptop is an ideal place to sleep. Particularly important was my daughter, Rose Adler, who helped prepare some of the images. A number of students provided help in researching some of the topics: Kristopher Few, Mary Rothermal, Sarah Shields, Alecia Czapski and (between National Guard duties) Taylor Janus. I also thank Dawn Eurich, archivist at the Detroit Public Library, for help in locating various letters and documents. Doug Bancroft of the Port Huron Historical Museum provided both information and photographs, as did Tim Hickey and Sue Child from Lakeside Cemetery in that city. All were helpful in tracking down information.

Introduction

Prior to 2010, if one asked the average person what they knew about cholera, at best the answer would probably be that it was some nineteenth century disease that we no longer have to fear. As of the first years of the twenty-first century, cholera as an epidemic disease has largely disappeared from Canada and the United States, at least in our collective memory. We have been fortunate. According to statistics released by the Centers for Disease Control and Prevention, between 1995 and 2000, 61 cases of cholera were reported in the United States, with a single death.[1] All cases were associated with a single strain of the bacterium *Vibrio cholerae* O1, which suggested a common source, or at least sources infected with the strain prevalent during this time. Most cases were associated with contaminated seafood.

A more significant outbreak took place in the United States during the first five years of the 1990s. One hundred ninety-five cases were reported during those years, nearly 70 percent of which had originated in South America; the numbers included 75 victims arriving on a single airliner from Peru. This outbreak involved a different strain of the organism from that described above, *Vibrio cholerae* O139, the prevailing strain in what has been recognized as the latest cholera pandemic. This last pandemic likely originated, as did the previous worldwide pandemics, from regions of Asia. However, unlike previous outbreaks, this one did not begin in India.

In January 2010 a devastating earthquake rocked large portions of Haiti, killing an estimated 200,000 persons and displacing over one million. Access to proper sanitation facilities and clean water were among the first challenges the survivors faced. By October 2010 the first cases of severe diarrhea were reported to health authorities, and shortly afterwards the cause of the diarrhea was identified as the bacterium *Vibrio cholerae*: cholera. By the time Haitian authorities, aided by the interna-

Introduction

tional community, brought the outbreak under control, over 470,000 cases had been reported, with a mortality rate of approximately 14 percent; once proper medical facilities were set up, the mortality rate dropped below 1 percent.[2]

While the scope of the tragedy associated with the earthquake itself—the enormous death toll, the loss of infrastructure in what was already a poverty-stricken country—staggers the modern mind, the outbreak of cholera that occurred in the aftermath is a story in itself. First, despite the (relatively few) cases that have appeared in the United States, an appearance largely forgotten in most of North America, we are reminded that what had been a devastating nineteenth century disease remains endemic in portions of Latin and South America. As recently as 1995 nearly 90,000 cases of the disease were reported in northern South America.[3] Between 1991 and 1993 nearly one million cases were reported in Latin America, though with a case fatality rate below 1 percent thanks to modern methods of treatment. This was likely the source for the small outbreak in the United States during these years.

The second lesson from this tragedy is that, unlike the situation with the nineteenth century pandemics, we know precisely the etiological agent behind the disease, and the mechanism by which cholera is transmitted: an average sized (1 micrometer in length) bacillus with a slight curve to its shape—hence the designation of "comma-bacillus." We know how the disease is transmitted: generally through water supplies contaminated with sewage, the solution to the problem being supplying fresh water to the population, or at least water that has been properly treated to eliminate this organism as well as others associated with waterborne disease. While any deaths due to cholera are to be regretted, the relatively low mortality rate also reflected both the existence of antibiotics that can effectively treat the illness if provided early enough, and the recognition that, while the vibrio toxin is the precise cause of the severe water loss, death can be averted by timely infusion, either orally or through transfusion, of water and physiological concentrations of salts.

Such was not always the case. The first cholera pandemic took place roughly between 1817 and 1826, beginning in the Ganges River delta of India and spreading throughout the region as far as Indonesia and even into portions of Eastern Europe. Mortality was in the hundreds of thou-

Introduction

sands, including some 10,000 British troops occupying the colony. By 1826 the disease had disappeared in much of the world, continuing only in endemic pockets that remained in India.

The second pandemic began in India in 1829, spreading through portions of Russia as well as Egypt, reaching the European continent the following year. Irish immigrants brought the disease to Lower Canada, from where it spread to Buffalo and ultimately through the Great Lakes region (including Detroit) and into what is now the Midwest. By 1834 cholera reached the Pacific. By the time the second pandemic was finished, ca. 1851, over 500,000 deaths, mostly in Europe, were left in its wake.

The third pandemic, beginning about 1852 in India and lasting the remainder of that decade, spread through much of Asia—Russia was particularly devastated, with over one million deaths—and into Europe and ultimately North America. It was this outbreak in London from which John Snow, as described later, obtained much of the information for his epidemiological studies. A minimum of several million deaths can be attributed to this pandemic, the most severe of the seven.

The fourth pandemic started in 1863. Originating, like the third, in the Bengal region of India, it was carried by Indian Muslims through the Middle East on the journey to Mecca. An estimated 30,000 persons on the *hajj* died from the disease, one-third of the total number of pilgrims. By 1879 the outbreak had claimed several hundred thousand victims.

The fifth pandemic, again originating in the Bengal region, began about 1881 and spread through much of Asia and Europe, killing over 200,000 Russians by the end of the outbreak in 1896. Nearly 60,000 persons died in Egypt. It was this outbreak, likely originating with English ships traveling from India through the recently opened Suez Canal, that resulted in three European commissions coming to Egypt to investigate the cause of the epidemic there. One of these, the German commission headed by Dr. Robert Koch, subsequently traveled to India, where Koch isolated and identified the etiological agent.

The sixth pandemic began about 1899, again in India, and by the time it was finished about 1923 had claimed nearly 500,000 victims in Russia and nearly one million in India. Europe and the rest of the West were largely spared from this outbreak, having instituted proper sani-

Introduction

tation procedures necessary to contain or prevent the disease. The United States was spared from the outbreak by instituting quarantine measures on several ships arriving from Naples and other ports in Italy and which contained passengers infected with cholera.[4]

The seventh, and what is considered by some to be the last, or at least latest, pandemic originated in Indonesia, unlike the previous six which began in India. It spread through portions of Pakistan, India, Russia and portions of Africa. Contemporary knowledge of sanitation helped limit the outbreak. Some consider the appearance of the new O139 strain, which first appeared in Asia in 1992, to actually represent an eighth pandemic.

But the subject of much of this history is primarily the story as it affected Detroit. While the disease would likely have ultimately spread by steamboat or other forms of shipping down the Great Lakes anyway, the 1832 epidemic in Detroit resulted from the movement of American troops under the command of General Winfield Scott, assigned the goal of suppressing the Native American uprising in regions of present-day Indiana and Illinois. Scott's men were exposed on the way, likely while in either New York City or Buffalo, and carried the contagion with them through much of what was then Michigan Territory.

The disease, which now became truly endemic to midwestern America, would periodically reappear in Detroit during the next three to four decades. The cause of the disease would remain a mystery during much of this time, being ascribed not only to lack of sanitation, but to the presence of lower classes of society; it was considered a poor man's disease, with this portion of society blamed as the source. No treatment was known, though as we see, there was no shortage of imagination as to how it might be treated; among this author's favorite remedies was the injection of ether.

The story of cholera in this book ends with the subsequent identification of a bacillus as the etiological agent of the disease, and an understanding of the nature of the pathology. During the 1890s the first effective vaccine was produced; that story is touched on as well. The isolation of the vibrio, first by the Italian physician Filippo Pacini, who was largely forgotten in his time, and then by Robert Koch, engendered its own dramatic story. In the present day the concept of an infectious origin to most illnesses—a bacterium or virus and sometimes some other form

Introduction

of parasite — has become second nature. The news in recent months (spring and summer 2012) has included the outbreak of a respiratory disease among campers in Yellowstone Park; a form of hantavirus was quickly identified. The etiological agent of an illness that killed more than 60 Cambodian children was quickly identified as a strain of the common hand, foot and mouth disease virus. The last time this author remembers a disease outbreak being ascribed to some mysterious miasma in the air was the Legionnaire's Disease outbreak in 1976 in Philadelphia; the agent there turned out to be a common soil bacterium.

This was not always the case with cholera, even after the germ theory of disease had been developed to explain the role of a living etiological agent and the disease it engendered. Two schools of thought, each supported by prominent physicians and scientists of the time, attempted to explain the underlying basis of the disease. The "contagionists" argued in favor of a specific etiological agent, using the example of outbreaks that followed the movement of peoples along trade or transportation routes. The challenge was explaining why cholera did not appear everywhere, or why medical personnel rarely became infected. The "miasmatists" believed the origin was outside the body, that it was endemic to the region in which cholera appeared. They blamed "vapors," odors of putrefaction that arose from the soil. The only way a person could protect himself was to aerate the soil in some fashion, or in the extreme, make his home airtight.[5]

Ultimately Koch and the "contagionists" were proven correct. Even so, some of the proponents of the miasma hypothesis did not go quietly. Max von Pettenkofer, among the most noted of the nineteenth century German scientists and physicians and a firm opponent of Koch's ideas on contagion, went so far as to drink a sample of the cholera bacillus. Fortunately for von Pettenkofer he suffered no significant ill effects. Fortunately for posterity, his timing was such that by then the infectious nature of cholera was largely accepted.

This book attempts to straddle two fields of interest: a medical story associated with Detroit as well as surrounding regions in what was initially the Territory of Michigan, and then the state of Michigan, and a medical history of a relatively modern disease, given the caveat that we begin in 1817. Cholera was not the only such waterborne disease in Detroit during these years, nor even the most common. But certain char-

Introduction

acteristics, most notably its explosive nature in the individual, set it apart from typhoid and dysentery. The latter two were so common that they were considered endemic, part of the "background," if you will, of living in a city. In contrast, between outbreaks, cholera was relatively rare. Its appearance during the described epidemics resulted in a profound change in the medical structure of the city, to say nothing of the local fame it brought to individuals such as Gabriel Richard and Martin Kundig, the former a victim of the disease.

The audience includes, but is not limited to, those with an intimate knowledge of Detroit and the pattern of its downtown. With the exception of the freeways ubiquitous in every city today, the layout of its downtown streets differs little today from that which existed in 1832, or for that matter, in 1870; anyone who attempts to drive through the inner city would certainly agree. But Detroit did not exist in a vacuum. Cholera first entered the United States in both Buffalo and New York City in 1832. New York City would continue as the focal point for the disease in later years. It was the outbreak and spread from Buffalo that particularly piqued my interest, as it overlapped with another of my hobbies, military history. The backdrop to the 1832 outbreak in the Midwest was the Black Hawk War, then raging in what are now portions of Illinois and Wisconsin. The troops sent from Virginia passed through both New York City and Buffalo, becoming exposed and ultimately transporting, along with their weapons, the cholera bacilli.

I have attempted to avoid a dry description of the history, despite the extensive citations, by limiting the medical jargon except where I feel necessary. I have also attempted to present the human aspect, examining the lives of individuals with something more than clinical interest. Anecdotes and trivia are included as they relate to the larger story. Extensive numbers of quotes from letters or writings, generally not found in a standard medical or history course, are presented so the reader can understand the thinking or reasoning as the contemporary writer observed or addressed a problem. In like manner, I have quoted extensively from the media or other personal accounts of the time. In some writings the underlying fear becomes apparent. After all, this was not the only illness faced by the people of the time; enteric illnesses such as typhoid and dysentery were endemic to most major cities. Where cholera differed from the other extant infectious diseases was in its explosive nature. Symptoms began as an intestinal upset or mild diarrhea; within a few hours the victim could be nearly drained of fluid as he or she faced a likely fatal outcome. As we now understand, rapid replacement of fluids is generally an effective treatment given the localized nature of the disease within the body; such knowledge was not available in the nineteenth century.

Snippets of the story can be found elsewhere in histories of Detroit; such sources are acknowledged when they were used. But I have found many of these sources were incomplete and sometimes inaccurate. Where only a last name might be reported in the historical accounts of books or articles, I attempted to locate more detailed information about the individual. In most cases I was successful. There were conflicting accounts in some cases; original sources, often newspaper accounts, provided more details and sometimes more accurate information.

1

From India to America

Cholera morbus, literally the "disease cholera." The name itself is ancient, dating at least to Hippocrates (ca. 5th century B.C.E.) and of unclear origin. The term is included among the four humors of Hippocratic medicine: sanguis (blood), melancholia (black bile), phlegm (phlegm) and cholera (yellow bile). The term may have been based upon the jaundice associated with a number of diarrheic diseases, or even the yellowish serum observed when blood is clotted, as suggested by Robert Fahraeus.[1] Others suggested it referred to the Greek term *cholera* as it applied to the gutter associated with a roof, reflecting intestinal discharges "flowing as from a spout."[2] Regardless, the disease we moderns call cholera was likely described at least 2,500 years ago. In their history of the disease, Barua and Greenough note that the word *visuchika* in Sanskrit literature may be a description of severe diarrhea associated with cholera. This interpretation is not universal.[3] Certainly the clinical description of the ailment as recounted by Barua from several sources is of an illness that resembles modern cholera: "matters collected in the stomach escape by vomiting, and the fluid matters in the belly and intestines run through by the lower passage. What is first vomited is like water, but what passes by stool is stercoraceous [fecal] and of ill odour.... But what is washed away is first like phlegm, afterwards like bile."[4] The reader understands the general picture. However, the possible epidemic nature of the illness is unclear from the sources. What could be interpreted as a description of cholera also fits the clinical description of numerous gastrointestinal diseases, either dysentery or viral in origin. The term *cholera* is found in the writings of Hippocrates, though his description of "dry cholera" is more of flatulence than the clinical illness: "the belly is distended with wind, there is rumbling in the bowels," and constipation rather than diarrhea is noted.[5] Perhaps a more accurate description by Hippocrates of what could truly be cholera followed: "At

Athens a man was seized with cholera. He vomited and was purged and in pain, and neither the purging nor the vomiting could be stopped; and his voiced failed him, and he could not be moved from his bed, and his eyes were dark and hollow, and spasms from the stomach held him, and hiccup from the bowels. He was forced to drink, and the two (vomiting and purging) were stopped, but he became cold."[6] Cholera? Perhaps. Dysentery or other form of gastrointestinal illness? Possibly. But Hippocrates provided vivid descriptions of a variety of similar diarrheic illnesses.[7]

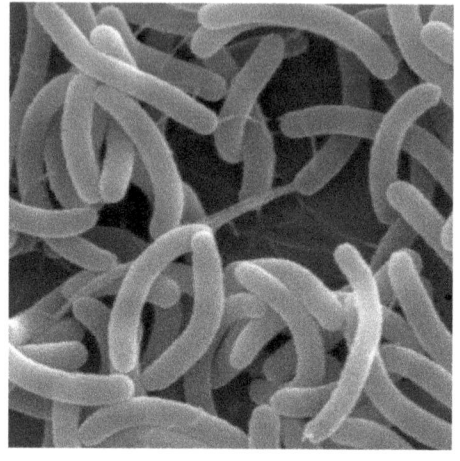

Electron microscopic image of *Vibrio cholerae*. Note the "comma" shape of the organism (courtesy Louisa Howard, Dartmouth College).

What is clear from history is that the first significant change from a localized disease clearly endemic to the Ganges River region on the Indian subcontinent to a European (and ultimately transatlantic) pandemic of cholera first began in 1817.[8] The outbreak of what became known as Asiatic cholera that year became the first of seven major pandemics to take place during the ensuing two centuries. From 1817 to 1823 the disease spread through much of Southeast Asia, parts of southern Russia, China and Japan and into the Middle East. Western Europe and England were spared—this time. The reasons for the outbreak during that period are to a significant degree reflected by the issues of our own times—a developing global economy, albeit an 1817 version, politics and military adventures. One possibility sometimes overlooked is the appearance of a new, more virulent strain of the organism. British physician Sidney Selwyn argued in favor of this hypothesis, based primarily upon the supposition that "cholera is a very young disease" and that "before 1781 there were no authenticated epidemics of true 'Asiatic cholera'—with profuse vomiting and rice-water stools." The appearance of these new symptoms "heralded the triumphal progress of true cholera beginning in Jessore [perhaps due to contaminated rice], near Calcutta, in 1817 when the first pandemic set out."[9] Reference to the year 1781 is included since it marked the first major outbreak among British troops located in India, sickening perhaps 500 men.[10]

Two major factors in 1817 contributed to the spread of the disease, which ultimately culminated in what became known as The First Pandemic. First was the movement of traders, both east and west. India was one of Great Britain's largest markets, and though trade in cotton and other textiles became increasingly one-sided by the 19th century as import duties protected British industries, for a time India provided a significant proportion of such goods imported into Britain. Shipping routes carried sailors and passengers to the Arabian Peninsula and beyond. Pilgrims likely spread the disease from Jessore to the larger cities as well. By the 1820s cholera had spread north and east to China and Japan. Meanwhile the British army was tied up in one of its many wars in Afghanistan and elsewhere on the Indian subcontinent, and was having to address its own encounters with the disease in September 1817:

> However well chosen might be the position of the Marquis of Hastings' headquarters on the banks of the Sind [northern India] ... it was found necessary to relinquish it on account of a dreadful pestilence which ravaged the camp of the centre Division. This destructive disease, since denominated cholera spasmodic, advanced from the countries about the head of the bay where it made its first appearance, and, almost as soon as the troops began to move, was felt on the Jumnah.... The march of the troops was strewed with the victims of this malady, which latterly attacked the Europeans, though the natives, from their habit of low diet, appeared most exposed to it.

Of the latter, 200 and upwards are said to have died in one day.[11] The case fatality rates were likely higher among the British troops, though specific numbers were not provided. As many as 10,000 British soldiers may have succumbed.[12] The Afghans and Nepalese opposing the British and their native allies may have carried the disease first into Burma and ultimately to Java and Japan. At the same time, British warships carrying troops infected with the disease brought it to Muscat in Oran on the southeastern portion of the Arabian Peninsula. The British were there ostensibly to deal with the slave trade, though their intervention had as much to do with removal of the Wahhabi sect then in power and the agreement for a "General Treaty of Peace." Shortly after the British arrival, a cholera epidemic left 10,000 deaths in its wake.[13] Despite the spread of the disease north into present-day Syria and Iraq, Europe was largely spared at that time. Some professed that the reason cholera did not enter England or the continent was the "superior British way of life."[14]

Europe, and ultimately both North and South America, were not as fortunate with the spread of the second cholera pandemic. The second pandemic began in the same region of the Ganges as did the first, about 1828, and began its spread through largely the same mechanisms, following trade routes throughout India into China and Russia, and eventually west by 1831 into present day Poland and Finland. The appearance in Finland the disease, spreading from present-day Poland, was most likely due to the presence of Polish troops then in revolt against the Russian empire.[15]

Cholera reached both Vienna and Berlin by mid–1831 and Paris by early 1832. As many as 20,000 persons may have died in Paris; 96 of the first 98 cases proved fatal.[16] The port of Sunderland, a town of some 20,000 persons on the Durham coast about 12 miles from Newcastle, may have been the starting point for the English outbreak during October 1831. While introduction of cholera through Sunderland has been accepted as the mechanism by which the epidemic spread from Europe to England, the belief was not universal. At least one report suggested English men-of-war lying below London during the summer of 1831 may have carried passengers ill with cholera. The ships had embarked from Riga and elsewhere in Russia where outbreaks had taken place. Over 150 persons became ill with what was assumed to be cholera, likely caused by "a miasm radiating from the ships."[17]

Cholera then proceeded to move south to London early in 1832; over 6,000 persons died there.[18] Though sporadic cases had appeared in Sunderland during that summer, authorities largely ignored an outbreak that they considered as merely "common cholera." Consequently, quarantine regulations were ignored as ships routinely entered the harbor. Even when it had become clear that a cholera epidemic was taking place in Sunderland, medical authorities refused to recognize its severity and the potential for a national epidemic. In part this reflected increased pressure from the business community: "The coal-owners, coal-merchants and other traders declared aloud that the physicians, some of whom had seen the disease in India, had formed a rash and erroneous

1. From India to America

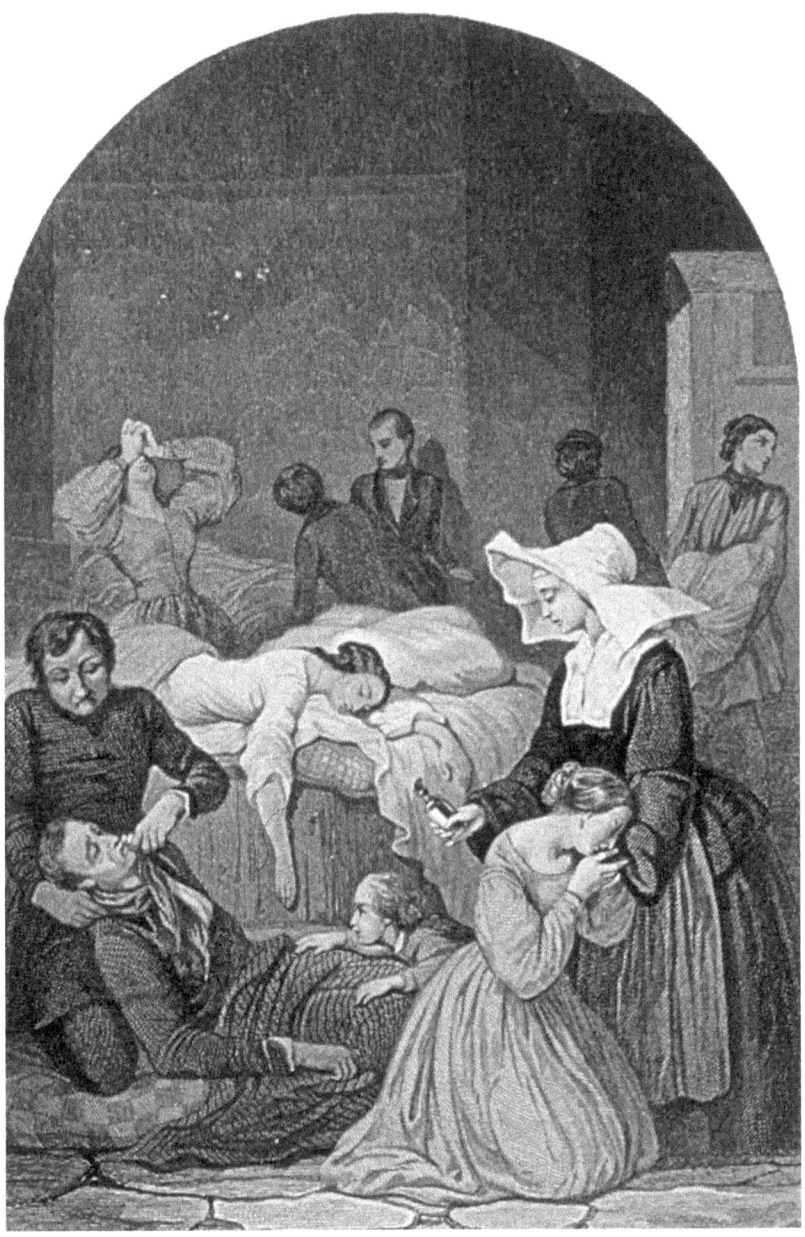

Cholera treatment during 1832 epidemic (image from the History of Medicine, National Library of Medicine).

judgment; that the first five cases were severe common cholera, and denied that it was by any chance imported. It was true that no crew members had yet died from the disease (October 26); it was also true that contaminated bed clothing was probably already on shore."[19] In some places wells and pump water were placed on streets in close proximity to sewer water. Even when the water had become impure and foul smelling, the significance of the odor was ignored.

Early in 1832 the disease appeared in Ireland, ultimately causing 25,000 deaths in what was then part of Great Britain.[20] The outbreak in Ireland during the spring and summer of 1832 could not be confined to the island given the increasing level of immigration to North America, and in particular immigration to the Canadian provinces. Conditions on passenger ships were appalling: "They travelled across the ocean in overcrowded ships in which they were forced to live in dreadful filth and squalor. The long and frequently treacherous Atlantic crossing meant that many in steerage spent from five to twelve weeks in dark, dank, cramped, unsanitary holds which were described by one traveler as filthy, filled with a fetid stench and containing hundreds huddled together like animals."[21] Adults in steerage were legally allowed a maximum of approximately 1.5 square yards of space. Even this was often ignored, as owners crammed as many passengers as possible on their ships.

The initial destinations for passengers embarking for Canada in the 1830s were the towns of Montreal and Quebec, both crowded and largely unsanitary. The arrival of tens of thousands of immigrants from Europe greatly exacerbated the problems. In June 1832 alone, 10,600 immigrants arrived in Quebec City, overwhelming whatever facilities existed for the influx of people.[22] In order to protect the populations from the threat of cholera arriving with immigrants, a quarantine station was established on the uninhabited island of island of Gross Isle in February. The extensive timber growing on the island was cut to supply wood for the hospital and administration buildings. The island was located in an advantageous spot, situated some 30 miles north (downstream) of Quebec City. Ships coming upriver were required to stop for inspection by local health officers, and any ships that had embarked from ports in which cholera was present — in 1832 meaning almost any departures from Europe or England — had to remain for a minimum of three days' quarantine. A military post was placed on the island to enforce the measure, the first

1. From India to America

quarantine act established in the Canadian province. All passengers had to clean themselves. If any cases of cholera were onboard, the ship underwent an additional 15-day quarantine.[23] Any passengers diagnosed with cholera spent three weeks convalescing in the hospital wards. Enforcement was sporadic. In Montreal not even these precautions were enacted.

The arrival of thousands of immigrants each week quickly overwhelmed the inspection facilities, with over 7100 persons passing through Grosse Isle alone from June 2 to 5.[24] Even with the best intentions on the part of the health officers, as well as a second inspection at the landing in Quebec, some ships passed without proper quarantine. At least three ships arriving from Ireland during April and May carried passengers with the disease; from 10 to 20 deaths were reported on each ship. Cholera arrived on the mainland of Canada in early June of that year, nearly simultaneously at both Montreal and Quebec City.[25] The first evidence in Quebec of a cholera outbreak came in that first week of June. Passengers on the ship *Carricks*, which had originated from Dublin and docked on June 3, had been reported as carrying the disease; approximately 45 of 145 passengers, a number that included the cabin boy, had died and been buried at sea. The *Carricks* might even have been considered cursed. In 1847, while carrying Irish immigrants fleeing the potato famine, it sank off the Gaspé Peninsula in the St. Lawrence River. Eighty-seven of the 187 passengers were drowned. The ship's bell can be found in a local church, next to a monument remembering the victims of the wreck.

Quarantine of passengers from infected ships was barely practiced. The only attempt at separation that took place was to segregate those persons who actually showed symptoms of disease from those who were not ill, or at least had not yet shown any symptoms. These passengers were not held and were simply allowed to proceed to their destination. Despite initial denials by officers with the Board of Health that there was cholera in Quebec, within the first week after the initial reported case, over 160 persons had died from the disease. The assumption was that either infected passengers or contaminated clothing was the source. Nor would cholera be confined to Quebec. A second ship, *Voyageur*, "a pestilent steamer owned by speculators whose morality lay in profit,"[26] was also reported to carry infected passengers who had landed at Quebec, and was even then on its way to Montreal. At least one passenger, Charles Vasseur, died.[27]

Within a week, over 160 persons succumbed to the disease in Quebec City. The outbreak began there at a boarding house on Champlain Street, "a house so filthy that it was described as a public nuisance."[28] The death toll averaged over 100 each day for a week before beginning its decline.

The *Voyageur* departed from Quebec City on June 7. At least two passengers were reported to have become ill on the way to Montreal: John Kerr, an immigrant from Derryaghy, Ireland, and a second man from Ireland, John McKee. Kerr died en route and McKee shortly after being brought ashore in Montreal.

The deaths of Kerr and McKee not only introduced cholera into the town of Montreal; the deaths created a panic among the citizenry: "Women with terror in their countenances, and many of them weeping were to be seen on every Street; ... carts with coffins containing dead bodies, each occupied with four or five persons were passing frequently.... Business seemed paralysed ... and many of our citizens left town, and a fine panic of almost indescribable nature seemed to have taken hold of the whole body of citizens."[29] While the disease made its first appearance in the poorer neighborhoods, those without proper sewage or sanitation, it quickly spread into even the "better" areas of the town. The newspaper *La Minerve* eventually acknowledged the presence of the disease, though it attempted to warn the citizenry against panic: "Since Monday morning Montreal is in turmoil and the alarm is growing every minute. There is no longer doubt that cholera is present. We recommend that the public observe strictly the Regulations of the Board of Health.... There is no use in becoming alarmed. When the illness appears one must see a doctor and follow his instructions. The apothecaries have all the necessary remedies in stock and their prices are affordable to all pocketbooks."[30] The preventives used by the authorities reflected the belief that cholera was transmitted through the air, as some form of miasma. Tar was burned in the hope that the smoke would purify the air and destroy the source of the disease, a common method of perceived preventive. The belief that the odors of the dead were related to the spread of cholera was not new; attempts to prevent the spread of what was called "The Great Mortality," the plague, during the Middle Ages often utilized pleasant-smelling vapors. Cannon were fired, perhaps in the hope they could "scare" the agent. More likely this was based on the belief that doing something, anything, was better than simply waiting. One might even blame the weather: "It is a singular fact that for about forty days previous to the appearance of the Cholera at Quebec, the wind had blown from the east; and it is inferred that the poison in the European atmosphere which generated the disease, has thus been communicated to this continent."[31]

By the end of June over 1,050 persons had died, the victims being primarily among the poor and immigrant population of the town. As was frequently the case, the interpretation among the upper classes was that cholera, if not caused directly by intemperance and "filthy habits," was at least associated with such behaviors. They were soon proven wrong, as the disease shortly demonstrated that it was no respecter of social class. Louis Lagueux, a member of the Quebec parliament, as well as Judge Jean Thomas Taschereau each fell victim to the disease. Lagueux had even mocked the ill, that they "should stand it *en grenadier* (as a soldier)."[32] As an eye witness, merchant Alexander Hart, related, "None of us go into town anymore. Many are moving into the country. Yesterday thirty-four corpses passed our house. Today, twenty-three ... not counting those in the old burial ground or in the Catholic ground. Twelve carts are employed by the Board of Health to carry away the dead who are interred without prayers."[33] By the time the disease had run its course in Montreal some 2,000 persons had died.

Cholera did not remain within the confines of the larger towns. As citizens attempted to flee the outbreak they carried the disease with them. The Montreal Board of Health had suggested that somehow the location of Montreal, "the abundance of low and marshy land, with its stagnant water filled with all the elements of miasma (pestilential effluvia) and the large number of vacant lots covered with rotting animal and vegetable matter," might be at fault.[34] But cholera began to appear even in small towns and villages. Between June 16 and June 20 cholera broke out in Prescott, Brockville and Kingston, all among persons who had fled Montreal. Some of those fleeing the outbreak crossed the St. Lawrence, bringing cholera into New York State. On June 13, "an emigrant recently from Montreal, died of cholera at Burlington, and on the 18th a female, who was addicted to intemperance, died of the same disease." That same day "an emigrant who had left Montreal on the 8th died of cholera at Plattsburg. He had been exposed to wet and cold, and was imprudent in diet. Several other cases occurred among residents of a filthy portion of the village [Plattsburg]; they were all persons of irregular habits."[35] Regardless of who brought the disease, and whatever reason could be found to blame the victim, cholera had crossed the border into the United States.

2

Cholera Crosses the Border

Given the level of the outbreak in towns along the St. Lawrence River in Lower Canada as the disease spread from Montreal and Quebec, the near impossibility of effective quarantine measures, and the ready movement of the populations in both directions, it was inevitable that the outbreak would eventually cross the river into the United States. In June 1832 the first cases appeared along the border region of New York State. The first confirmed death from cholera was that of a man who, on the 8th of that month, had been in Montreal. On June 13 he died in Plattsburg, New York. It was pointed out that he was a man "imprudent in diet," while other persons in the "filthy portion of the village and "of irregular habits" also contracted the disease.[1] The description of the man and the implication that his social status and personal habits had played a role in contracting the disease was obviously meant to assure other residents of the town that they had little to fear, as long as they did not associate with that class of people. Social class aside, it was obvious that cholera was spreading throughout the region in an indiscriminate fashion. That same day another former resident of Montreal succumbed to cholera in Burlington. During the week that followed, an increasing number of cases began to appear in towns within close proximity of the Canadian border: On June 14 a man who had recently spent several days in Montreal, and who had apparently been briefly hospitalized for undisclosed reasons at the time, developed the disease while traveling on the steamboat *Phoenix* on Lake Champlain. He was taken to White Hall at the southern end of the lake near the Vermont border, where he died the next day. He was described as being "very" intemperate. A porter on the same boat died on the 16th of June. The town of White Hall was quarantined following the appearance of these cases, resulting in several hundred emigrants being held in the town for several days.

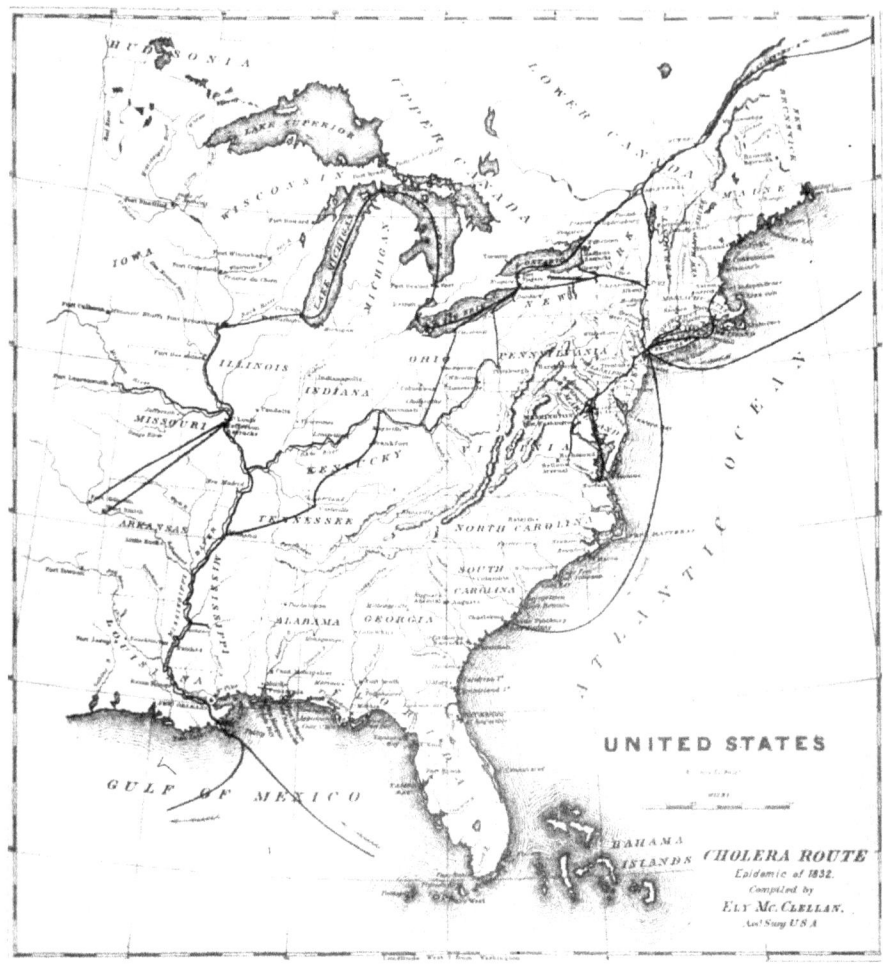

Path of the 1832 epidemic from Europe to Canada and ultimately throughout the western United States (image from the History of Medicine, National Library of Medicine).

It quickly became clear that the disease was spreading south from Montreal and Quebec City while following a route along Lake Champlain and the Champlain Canal, appearing in Mechanicsville and Rouse's Point the third week of June. The victim in Mechanicsville was an emigrant from Montreal, having departed from that city on June 11, five days before he died. Other towns and villages in both Upper Canada (Prescott,

Brockville and Kingston) as well as upper New York State described similar outbreaks; in Kingston alone during the period from mid–June to mid–July, 165 cases, with 52 deaths, were reported. Dr. Lewis Beck (1798–1853) had been appointed by New York governor Enos Throop in 1832 to "procure information in relation to the existence, progress, spread, origin, prevention and treatment of malignant or spasmodic cholera."[2] Beck was a logical choice for the assignment. He had received his medical degree in 1815, and eight years later moved to Albany, New York where he spent most of the remainder of his life. Though licensed to practice medicine, his major interest was the study of plants; during his lifetime Beck had positions as professor of botany, chemistry and natural history at various colleges in the state. He was also noted as the discoverer of several new species of plants.

In his role as advisor on cholera for the governor, Beck spent much of the year traveling throughout the state recording the story of the outbreak, which included not only the sites in which the disease appeared, but statistics related to the numbers of cases and the characteristics of the victims, many of whom he described as "filthy" or "intemperate." The final report was delivered to the governor in August 1832. In addition to the vivid description of the disease itself, Beck noted

> that the disease has generally passed from place to place along the main channels of communication. Wherever it has prevailed to any extent, the infected city or village appears to become a centre from which the disease is communicated to different places in the vicinity. Thus from Montreal and Quebec, as centres, it gradually spread into various parts of Canada, following the course of emigration. Cases also appeared on the line of our Northern canal, and at different points on Lake Champlain. In most of the villages on the Canadian side of the St. Lawrence, and of Lake Ontario, where the tide of emigration has been uninterrupted, the cholera has occurred; while on the American side, where, since the breaking out of the disease at Montreal, all communication with the Canadas has been stopped, not a case has been reported except at Ogdensburgh, and one or two other points on the St. Lawrence, where the intercourse could not be so completely interrupted.
>
> Again, when the disease was once located at Albany, boatmen and others leaving the city were attacked in various places, both on the line of the canal and elsewhere; and it appeared to radiate from this as a centre. The same fact has also been observed at New York, from which by travel the disease has been communicated to cities and villages in the vicinity, and even at some distance.[3]

Beck's report could be considered classic in its description of the spread of a disease from what later might be referred to as "point sources." In some respects it anticipated the later epidemiological study of cholera carried out by John Snow in London during the 1850s outbreaks in that city. Snow traced the origin at that time to contaminated water supplies. But Beck was incorrect in one interpretation of his data, believing that cholera was not a contagious disease, one certainly not contagious in the same manner as smallpox or measles. He based this belief on the seemingly unusual epidemiological characteristics of the outbreak, that attendants to cholera victims, particularly physicians, rarely developed the disease, and villages or towns in close physical or commercial proximities to where outbreaks were taking place did not always suffer from the presence of the disease. In their analysis of Beck's report, Ashleigh Tuite and colleagues suggested that the reason for Beck's reluctance to ascribe a contagious nature to the disease lay in the social and moral context of the period, rather than in any medical deficiencies on his part.[4] More specifically, since an apparently inordinate number of victims were those in the lower or "intemperate" classes, in Beck's view — and in the view of those in the contemporary evangelical fields as well — it was the absence of a proper moral character combined with poor personal habits that placed the person at increased risk of contracting the disease.

By June 30 the first cases were appearing in New York City, though it wasn't entirely clear whether the source was the movement of the disease south from Albany, or emigrants on ships arriving from Europe. It was reported that a "Dr. [Alexander] Vache stated that the ship *Henry IV* arrived in New York harbor, with cholera on board, in the latter part of June."[5] While Vache had been in New York at the time of the 1832 outbreak, he only provided this observation in 1850. The reason for the long delay is unclear, as is the accuracy of the date. What is known is that persons exposed to the disease not only remained within the city and its environs, but also began traveling to other regions of New York State: Albany, Rochester and even Buffalo. Evidence exists that Vache was correct in his implication that the outbreak in New York City was independent of that in Canada. Dr. John S. Westervelt, the first physician for the Port of New York, noted that emigrants arriving in infected ships were carrying the disease prior to outbreaks that may have originated elsewhere. Quarantine records for the city in the period covering April through June 1832 disappeared, while records outside of that period remained extant, lending credence to the belief that the outbreak was covered up.

Exposure of the citizens of Buffalo, then a city of over 10,000 persons, came from two directions: the east, particularly in travelers following the Erie Canal, as well as from both Lower and Upper Canada, via persons crossing the river. Buffalo had originated as a trading post in the late 18th century. The town had been burned by the British during the War of 1812 and had barely begun to recover even a decade later. However, its location near the terminus of the Erie Canal, opened in 1825, had resulted in the small village suddenly taking on the appearance of a boom town; the population increased from some 2,500 persons in 1825 to approximately 10,000 by the time of the 1832 outbreak.[6] The sudden growth was accompanied by many of the "features" associated with a lack of understanding of public health, poor sanitation among them, and with the development of a less-than-desirable class of citizens who patronized saloons, gambling dens and prostitutes. The area surrounding the canal was a particularly wild place, with one witness estimating that "sixty percent of the buildings on both sides of Canal Street from Erie Street to Commercial were houses of prostitution, thirty percent were saloons, and ten percent grocery stores" or legitimate businesses.[7] Both human and animal waste, as well as the occasional human body, were tossed into the canal. The odor was such that locals were often ill simply from the smell. Typhoid fever was only one of a number of diseases commonly associated with conditions euphemistically called unsanitary. It is no surprise that the introduction of cholera from across the border would result in the rapid establishment and spread of the disease.

The outbreak of cholera in Buffalo during the 1832 epidemic was particularly hard, sparing neither the well-to-do nor the poor. Even those who were seemingly perfectly healthy were at risk—feeling fine in the morning and dead by that night was a common description of the course of the illness. The administrative Common Council did what it could. Once it became clear the disease had appeared, the council established a board of health, composed of Roswell Haskins, a local printer and bookbinder, attorney Dyre Tillinghast, Lewis F. Allen and the presiding member, Dr. Ebenezer Johnson, who had also been elected as the first mayor of the city.[8] Assisting the Board was the local undertaker, Loring Pierce, and health adviser Dr. John Marshall.

The Board of Health met on a daily basis to discuss or propose procedures that might protect the town against the approaching epidemic. The most obvious measure was the institution of a quarantine:

> Steamboats were stopped on their entrances to the harbor until their passengers and crews had passed health inspection; stage coaches were stopped outside the city; canal boats were met below Black Rock[9] as they were coming to their destination, and country people kept at a safe distance outside by their own fears of contagion. Everybody but the reckless ones lived on half rations of food, so far as vegetables and fruits were concerned, and the most abstemious of all diluted their water with a modicum of what, by courtesy, was called "French brandy"; while the tipplers (and they were more than enough) held a prolonged saturnalia of bibulous indulgence.[10]

The first hospital, actually a former brick tavern called the McHose House, was established near Niagara and Ninth streets. In an ironic twist, Loring Pierce, the undertaker, was in charge of the arrangements for admission of cholera patients, and, presumably, removing the bodies of those who had died. Among the first such deaths was the chief nurse. To replace the nurse, Pierce hired a 25-year-old Irish woman, Bridget, who within several days also succumbed to the disease.

Among the victims were major figures in the newly incorporated city: Martin Chittenden, a local lawyer,[11] and District Attorney Henry White.[12] White had spent an afternoon at the local hotel. That evening he complained of not feeling well; by morning he was dead. Samuel Welch, in his history of the city, described the presence of "death carts," which roamed the city at night collecting the bodies of those who had died during the day. If there appeared to be a death in house, the driver would yell to the occupants, "Bring out your dead." The dead were quickly buried, often within an hour or two after collection.[13] Fear of the disease followed the victims to the grave. For a time, victims of cholera were not permitted burial in the primary cemetery laid out in the then-nearby village of New Amsterdam, and special burial sites were established.

As was the case in most places dealing with cholera outbreaks, neither the cause, prevention or treatment was understood. Remedies were almost quaint when compared with our understanding of the disease in modern times. Many persons wore bags of gum camphor around the neck, hoping to stave off the infection. At least one local remedy had its origins in an article published in the newspaper, the *New York Sun*, titled "The Sun Cholera Mixture": Equal parts tincture of opium, red pepper, rhubarb, essence peppermint, and spirits of camphor. The patient was to swallow 10 to 20 drops in several teaspoonfuls of water. The solution was not to be mixed with alcohol.[14]

The first confirmed case of cholera in Buffalo was on July 15 or 16. According to one report, the victim was "an Irish laborer, an habitual drunkard," who died within eight hours after symptoms developed[15]; again the disease was seen as, in part, a reflection of the social or personal habits of the victim. A separate description was more benign, making no reference to an Irish laborer: "The first case was in the person of a boatman on the canal who had been engaged in rafting lumber for three days previous."[16] It is not impossible that both descriptions represented the same individual, the point source of the epidemic, as epidemiology in a later century would describe the victim. However, it is more likely that the disease was present in the city even before this, as attested by a letter provided by a local physician, Cyrenius Chapin, to the Board of Health in Buffalo[17]: "To the Clerk of the Board of Health, Within the past 24 hours [i.e. July 12th] I have prescribed for the following patients, R.B. London, age 37 yrs.... His disease is cholera morbus. He is a man of intemperate habits."

What follows in Chapin's report is a description of six additional cases, four at the same house. All appeared to be convalescing at the time of this report. Clearly the cases reported on the 15th or 16th were not the first, and cholera was present in the city for at least the previous week. Chapin had been a lieutenant-colonel of volunteers during the War of 1812, leading a troop of some 50 riflemen against the British. He was eventually taken prisoner when Buffalo was captured by the British. At the time of the outbreak in Buffalo, Chapin was a well-respected physician over 60 years of age, who could be quite abrupt, a man who was not afraid to speak his mind. He did not take kindly to the requirement for submission of daily reports about progression of the disease to the Board of Health: "Why should I report my medical cases to a set of ignoramuses who don't know the cholera from whooping cough? No, I'll see 'em hanged first."[18] Chapin was eventually persuaded that discretion was preferable and subsequently did provide his reports, albeit with reluctance. Chapin's medical partner, Dr. Bryant Burwell, was a study in contrasts when comparing the two physicians. Burwell was a much more pleasant, less dictatorial individual, one who had no problem with submission of the requested reports.

Roswell Haskins, a member of the Board of Health, had duties that included the inspection of any ships entering the locks at Black Rock. One midnight when Haskins and other board members were on duty, four Canadian schooners appeared. The board rowed several small boats out to greet them, and when the boarding party appeared on deck the captains for each ship were called and told their respective ships would have to be inspected:

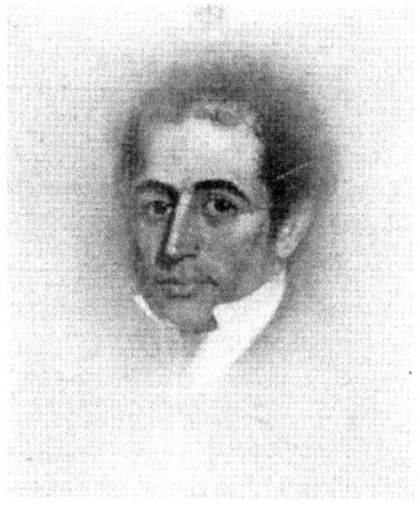

Marshall Chapin, twice mayor of Detroit (1831–1833), who held the position of city physician during the 1832 cholera outbreak.

> In no very decorous terms, [the captains] bade the invading party be gone. But this was of little use; the visitors were strong enough to protect themselves. The condition of the crew and passengers was ascertained to be free from disease, and the boats with their visitors on board returned to the wharf whence they started. On reaching the shore the party went to the tavern nearby, where some of them restored their wasted strength by imbibing a trifle of the "medicine" so frequently taken to "ward off the effects of frequent exposure." On this occasion, Haskins, who never touched a drop of spirits, not even wine, cider, or beer — "would as soon drink aqua fortis" [nitric acid mixed with water, used as a cleansing agent] as either — was profusely liberal in setting a decanter of brandy before the boatmen, telling them to take all they wanted.
>
> "Why Haskins," said Allen to him, "what does this mean? Your precept and example both are against all dram drinking, and here you are, giving the opportunity to let these men get drunk at their pleasure." "Can't help that," replied Haskins. "If these chaps hadn't expected a treat of this kind,

we might have stayed ashore instead of getting to their vessels, and I am not the one to balk their appetites. Taking the liquor is their affair, not mine."[19]

The cholera outbreak in Buffalo lasted some two months, during which approximately 250 persons became ill, and 120 deaths occurred.

The timing of the cholera outbreak in mid–July in Buffalo plays a significant role in the question of when and how American troops may have been exposed to the disease. Fighting had broken out in the West between the Sac and Fox natives and white settlers; the conflict subsequently became known as the Black Hawk War, named for Black Hawk, the leader of the Sac and Fox. President Andrew Jackson "had grown impatient at what he considered a policy of what he considered procrastination and conduct which he is said to have characterized as pusillanimous on the part of the volunteers." He ordered General Winfield Scott, hero of the War of 1812, "to take nine companies from the Atlantic coast, proceed to the seat of war and put an end to it."[20] Scott departed from Fortress Monroe on the Chesapeake Bay in eastern Virginia on June 28. The troops would travel to Buffalo by way of New York City, then sail from Buffalo down Lake Erie to Detroit and around the lakes to Chicago by way of Fort Mackinac and Lake Michigan.[21] Four steamboats, at a cost of $5,000, were chartered by the United States government in the beginning of July to transport the troops along with any needed provisions from Buffalo to Chicago: the *Henry Clay*, the *Superior*, the *Sheldon Thompson* and the *William Penn*.[22] Use of one of the ships, the *Henry Clay*, became problematic. Prior to its charter as a troop transport steamer, the *Henry Clay* had served as transport for emigrants from the east, some of whom had already been infected with cholera. On June 10 the boat had docked in Cleveland while carrying victims of the disease; five crewmen on the boat had reportedly died from the disease which appears to have subsequently entered the town. An epidemic broke out shortly afterwards in Cleveland, claiming 50 lives. The boat was fumigated in hopes of eliminating the cause of the outbreak and proceeded on to Buffalo.[23] The army medical officer traveling with Scott later confirmed the likely source of the outbreak on board the steamers: "At the time it was generally believed that the principle of infection existed in the steamboat in which the troops were conveyed from Buffalo to Detroit, the vessel having been employed in transporting crowds of *filthy* [italics added] emigrants westward from Montreal and Quebec. The *Henry Clay*, among the troops on board of which the disease also appeared, had been engaged in the same kind of service."[24]

On July 1, three companies of artillery and four companies composed largely of new recruits under the commands of Lieutenant-Colonel David E. Twiggs[25] and Brevet Major Matthew Mountjoy Payne (4th Regiment of Artillery),[26] a total approximating 400 troops, embarked on the *Henry Clay*.[27]

Scott, his staff, six companies of artillery that he had brought from Fortress Monroe, and two companies of infantry embarked on the *Sheldon Thompson* under the commands of Lieutenant-Colonel Abraham Eustis, Brevet Lieutenant-Colonel Ichabod Crane and Colonel William J. Worth.[28] The soldiers had been in New York City on June 23. On that date they departed for Albany, where they arrived the next day. The troops were then transported through the western canal and arrived in Buffalo at the end of the week. While officially cholera did not appear in New York City until after the troops had departed, the timing is close enough that one could make the argument that exposure had been simultaneous with their presence. Because of unexpected winds the *Henry Clay* remained docked in Buffalo until July 3. The first cases of cholera appeared on the boat the following evening, on the 4th, when a soldier "of intemperate habits, and who had been indisposed for several days, was seized with cholera, and died in nine hours. Another case occurred soon after."[29] Lewis Beck, in his report to the New York State Medical Society, had attempted to explain the appearance of cholera in victims who seemingly had minimal contact with the disease. Not only did cholera

Charles Gratiot, graduate of the United States Military Academy and chief engineer for General William Henry Harrison during the War of 1812. In 1814 he helped design the fort that was named in his honor (courtesy Port Huron Historical Museum).

2. Cholera Crosses the Border

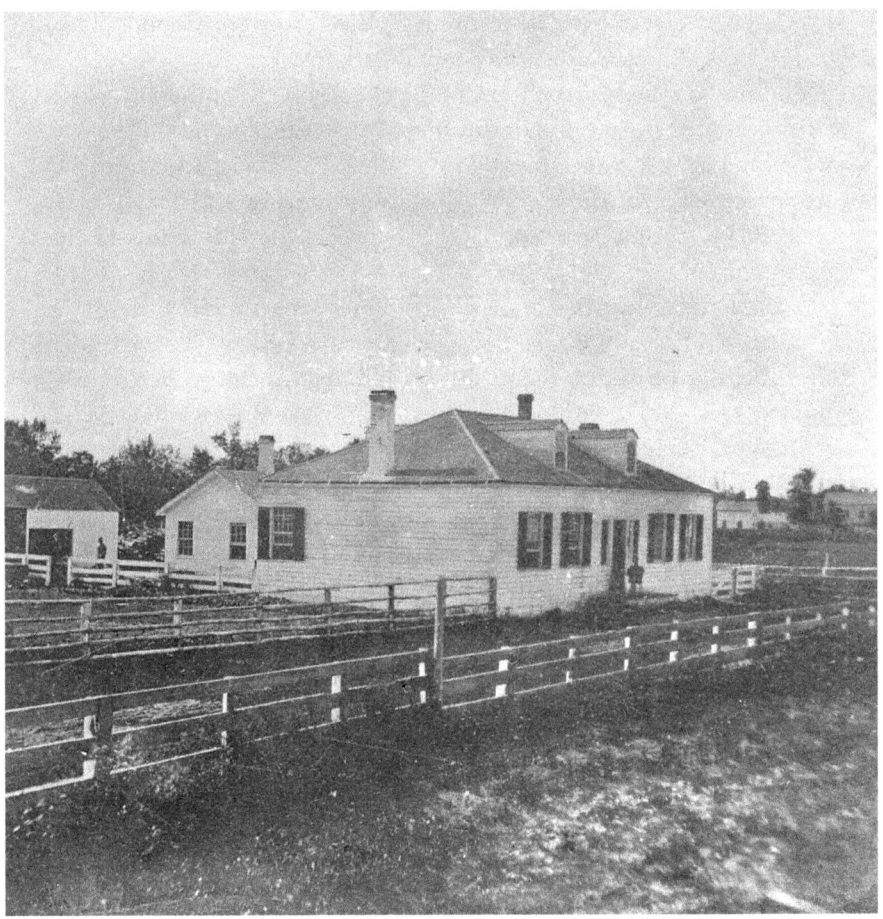

Fort Gratiot, ca. 1860s (courtesy Port Huron Historical Museum).

break out among troops once on board the steamers, but other cases were noted throughout the state. According to Beck, "The only general explanation that in my opinion can be offered is, that under the peculiar atmospheric constitution now so general, the disease may be brought out wherever a number of persons are crowded together for any length of time, especially when they are either filthy, badly fed or clothed, or intemperate."[30] Portions of Beck's description would certainly apply to at least a subset of the troops under Scott's command. It would be two decades before English physician John Snow provided convincing evidence that cholera was a disease resulting from exposure to contaminated water. Beck did touch on that possibility, however: "And I should also add, that the facts seem to warrant the conclusion, that the disease may be also excited by the effluvia given out by cholera patients, when other local causes favor its production."[31] Cholera had been present while the troops passed through New York City, was present in Buffalo concurrent with those troops, and had been present on the ship prior to their embarkation.

So the determination as to when and where the American troops were exposed is uncertain. While they may have been exposed during the days they spent in Buffalo, it is equally plausible they became infected either in New York City or in any of the towns they passed through on the way to Buffalo. The incubation period for cholera generally ranges from three to five days, long enough that troops might have been exposed either in New York City or in Buffalo, but less likely while on board the steamers which, while previously used to transport passengers who did develop cholera, had supposedly been cleaned. Regardless of where they had been exposed, troops on both the *Henry Clay* and *Sheldon Thompson* were now carrying the disease south from Buffalo through Lake Erie and were on their way to Fort Gratiot and, ultimately, Detroit.

Fort Gratiot

During the War of 1812, the conflict that played out in the West between Great Britain and its Native American allies and the young United States was often centered in the vicinity of Detroit and that portion of the Michigan Territory. While the origins of the war were complicated, the primary issues in the West centered on repeated incursions by Native American tribes, often encouraged by the British, in what was then considered the Northwest Territory — the present-day states of Indiana, Illinois, Wisconsin and Michigan, and until it became a state, Ohio. During the first months of 1812 President James Madison was pressured to create an army sufficient to defend the territory in the event of war, which was subsequently declared by the United States that June. William Hull, governor of the territory, was one of the few experienced officers available, having served honorably during the revolution a gen-

2. Cholera Crosses the Border

eration earlier, and was appointed by Madison as brigadier-general in charge of the territorial troops.

Hull was nearly 60 years old by then, and had never commanded a force of significant size. Not that such an army even existed in the West. The recruits available to Hull were few in number, primarily militia, and wholly inexperienced in the art of war. Early in July Hull and his men, numbering about 600 regulars and 1,700 militia, encamped at Fort Detroit, roughly the current site of downtown Detroit. Opposing them were approximately 500 British troops and native allies encamped across the Detroit River at Fort Amherstburg, south of present-day Windsor, Ontario. The British and natives were under the commands of General Isaac Brock and the Shawnee chief Tecumseh. Despite outnumbering their opponents, the Americans were short on food and supplies, suffered from low morale, and had few large guns to oppose the British. Fearing he was outnumbered, and recognizing his troops would likely be slaugh-

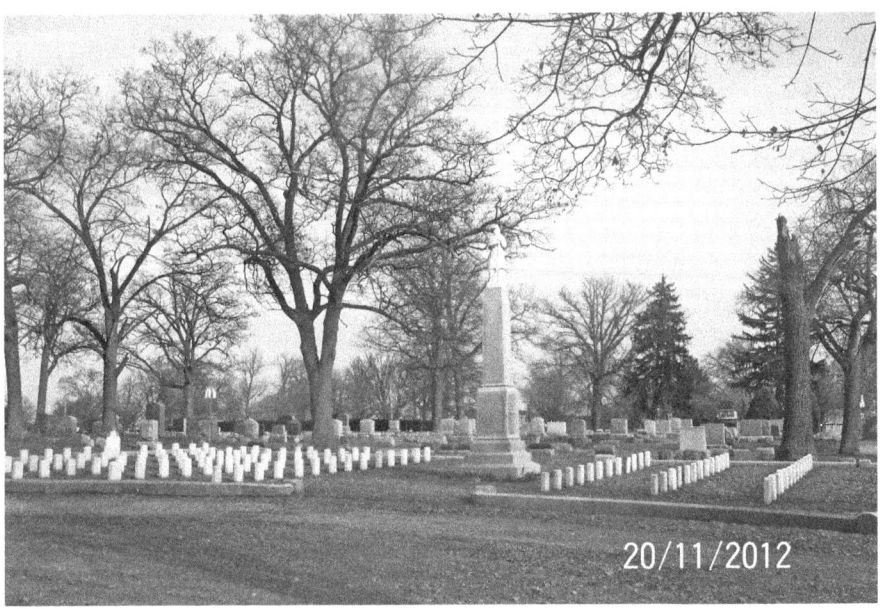

Lakeside Cemetery, graves of soldiers who died during the 1832 outbreak among General Scott's troops. The cemetery was established in 1877. In 1881, the remains of 135 soldiers buried at Fort Gratiot were re-interred here (courtesy Lakeside Cemetery, Port Huron).

tered if they did attempt to fight, Hull surrendered the town and fort in August. Detroit remained in British hands for another year until the American navy defeated the British in the Battle of Lake Erie, isolating Detroit and Fort Amherstburg and forcing the British to retreat.

The Treaty of Ghent, signed the day before Christmas in 1814, ended the war and returned to the United States any portions of the territory occupied by the British. The vulnerability of Detroit, and of the Great Lakes in general, resulted in the federal government's decision to establish a fort for the purpose of maintaining access to Lake Huron as well as providing a measure of protection against future incursions by Native Americans, many of whom, perhaps understandably, remained sympathetic to the British. Captain Charles Gratiot, a graduate of the United States Military Academy at West Point and a distinguished officer during the recent war in which he served as chief engineer to General William Henry Harrison, was ordered to oversee the construction of a fort north of the city of Detroit. In May 1814 Gratiot chose a site near that of a previous French fort, Fort St. Joseph, which had been abandoned during the previous century. The site was located on the western shore of the St. Clair River, ideally situated to guard the narrow entrance between the river and Lake Huron.

The fort consisted of a log and earthworks stockade, with an embankment on the western portion in anticipa-

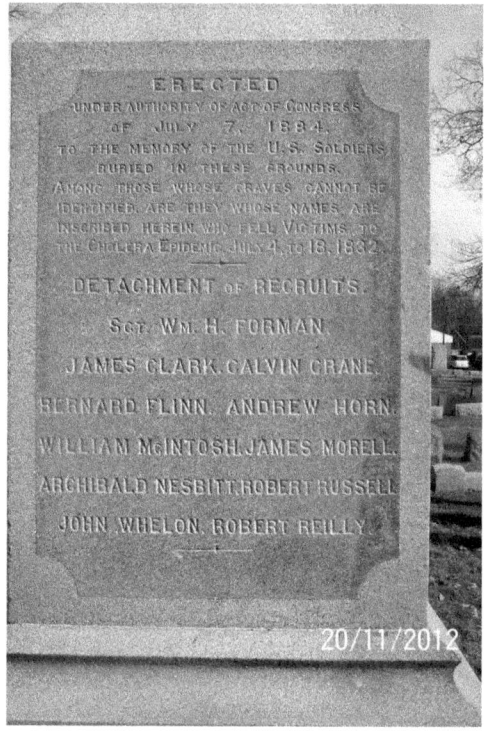

Lakeside Cemetery, monument honoring the soldiers who died during the 1832 outbreak among General Scott's troops whose remains could not be identified (courtesy Lakeside Cemetery, Port Huron).

2. Cholera Crosses the Border

tion of a native raid, and larger guns facing the river. A military road was constructed between the fort and town of Detroit, a distance of approximately 70 miles. Portions of the military road today are roughly represented by Gratiot Avenue, Michigan Route M3. A post road was also established between Detroit and Mt. Clemens, midway between the town and fort in 1820, the second such road in the territory.[32]

Fort Gratiot was occupied by American troops until 1821, at which time it became clear the fortification was no longer necessary, and it was abandoned. The fort was left to the elements and allowed to rot away. However, by 1828 the influx of thousands of settlers and lead-miners traveling into what is now southwestern Wisconsin resulted in renewed hostilities between the Americans and native peoples. As a consequence, all military installations along the shores of the lakes were reinforced. Fort Gratiot, by now existing primarily as mere earthworks, was rebuilt and re-established as a military post. The post road for the mails was also extended to Fort Gratiot. Because of the ever-present danger of shipwrecks on the shore, a lighthouse was constructed in 1825. The original lighthouse was extensively damaged by storms, and was rebuilt in 1829; the reconstructed lighthouse remains today.

Fort Gratiot was to play a significant role in the cholera epidemic that broke out in Detroit in 1832. As a fort, however, it was never subject to hostile fire, and once it became plain that its existence played no significant purpose, it was abandoned for the last time in 1879.[33]

3

Cholera Among the Troops

Certainly General Scott was aware of the potential danger of cholera infecting his troops. His army had passed through several areas of New York State in which the disease had already broken out: New York City and of course Buffalo. It bears repeating that the role of contaminated water was largely overlooked in 1832, and even though "animalcules" had been observed in contaminated waters since the development of the microscope, the germ theory of disease would not provide an explanation for the illness for another generation. So while the source of the outbreak was unknown, Scott still recognized that his own family was in danger as long as they remained in New York. Prior to traveling to Fort Monroe to take command of his regulars, Scott moved his family to West Point, site of the military academy, and placed his family in the hands of his friend Captain Ethan Allen Hitchcock, then commander of cadets at the academy. Scott returned to New York City and met with Dr. Thomas Gardner Mower to discuss the possibility that cholera could break out among his men, and how to deal with the disease if it did. Mower had been a leading army surgeon for nearly two decades and had served with the army as far back as the War of 1812. If any of Scott's extensive professional contacts would know how to deal with the disease it would be he. Mower provided Scott with information consistent with the knowledge extant in 1832. Treatment generally consisted of purging the victim, inducing evacuation of the bowel with administration of calomel, a mercury compound, which of course merely compounded the problem. If the patient still failed to recover, bleeding, blistering or the application of leeches were second options. Mustard plasters could be applied to the stomach. If all else failed, whiskey or laudanum (opium) could be administered. None of these time-honored remedies would alleviate the

3. Cholera Among the Troops

illness of course, but if nothing else the patient might be feeling no pain as he or she died. At least one physician had attempted, with some success, to revive patients through the injection of saline solutions: Dr. William O'Shaughnessy had been sent by the British Royal College of Surgeons in London to study the 1831 outbreak of cholera in Newcastle. O'Shaughnessy was cognizant of previous reports that as much as 30 percent of the fluid in blood was lost from the severe diarrhea as well as electrolytes, "denoting a great but variable deficiency of water in the blood in four malignant cholera cases; a total absence of carbonate of soda in two; and a remarkable diminution of the other saline ingredients. Again in the dejections passed by one of the patients ... we find preponderance of alkali, and we recover the other saline matters deficient in the blood." O'Shaughnessy proposed that as a means to remedy the loss that blood should be restored to its "natural specific gravity" and saline should be replaced. Among the physicians who carried out testing of O'Shaughnessy's ideas was Dr. Thomas Latta, considered the first major practitioner of fluid replacement. Despite his success with some patients, the treatment was ignored following Latta's death in 1833 from tuberculosis. Among the difficulties encountered by physicians in using this treatment was lack of standardization of saline solutions, plus the dangers of embolisms or phlebitis.[1] As with many new ideas however, the treatment would not be recognized or accepted for decades.

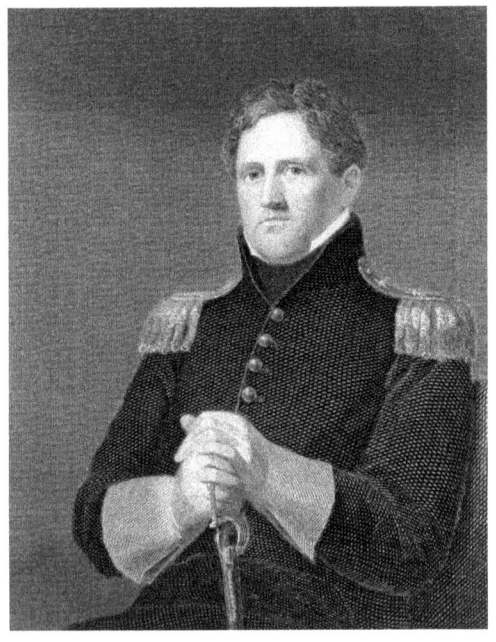

General Winfield Scott, hero of the War of 1812 and commanding officer of American troops during the Black Hawk War (courtesy United States Military Academy).

Following his meeting with Dr. Mower, Scott again reversed direction and traveled back up the Hudson to West Point where 29 cadets, constituting most of the graduating class of 1832 and out for adventure and some actual military experience, joined him for the trip to Buffalo. The sons of several prominent politicians and military figures were among these cadets, including Lieutenant George Crittenden, the son of Kentucky senator John Crittenden, and the sons of generals Jacob Brown, Robert Swartwout and Alexander Macomb.[2]

The military academy graduates were not assigned simply as observers. Among the orders General Scott issued were these:

> The graduates of the Military Academy [West Point], and officers who were on furlough, who have so gallantly volunteered their services for the campaign, will be distributed among the several battalions on their arrival at Chicago. In the mean time they will continue on duty with the troops to which they have been provisionally attached.... All officers are invited immediately to refresh their memories by reading over again the several articles Nos. 43 and 62 inclusive, under the head of "Economy of an army in the field, in the General Regulations for the Army."[3]

By the time Scott and his entourage reached Buffalo the four steamboats that he had chartered and his assigned troops were ready for embarkation to Detroit and their ultimate destination at Fort Dearborn/Chicago. Two of the steamboats, the *Henry Clay* and the *Sheldon Thompson*, would carry the officers, troops and equipment — Scott himself was on the *Henry Clay* along with his staff and the six companies of infantry originating at Fort Monroe as well as two companies from the 2nd Infantry — while the other two boats, the *William Penn* and the *Superior*, would transport provisions for the troops as well as other necessary supplies. The *William Penn* and *Superior* left several days after the *Henry Clay* and *Sheldon Thompson*. Unfavorable winds prevented the boats from leaving until July 3, at which date the trip began. Within a day cholera broke out among the seven companies commanded by Twiggs and Payne on the *Henry Clay* as the steamboat neared Detroit; two men were reported ill with the disease — one possibly being Lieutenant Joseph Clay — and subsequently died. The *Henry Clay* arrived at the dock in Detroit several hours ahead of the *Sheldon Thompson*.

Once they became aware of the outbreak of cholera on the approaching boat, the authorities in Detroit refused to allow the *Henry Clay* to remain at dock and ordered boat captain Walter Norton and his

3. Cholera Among the Troops

crew on the *Henry Clay* to continue up the river to Hog Island, where it could dock in a relatively isolated region apart from the town.[4] At the time the only medical officer on the *Clay* was Assistant Surgeon Robert E. Kerr. Once he learned of the outbreak on the *Clay* by July 5, Scott ordered surgeon and "medical director of the army in the field" Josiah Everett to assist Kerr in dealing with the outbreak. Everett's report to his superiors included the following item for July 7: "The troops and baggage, being landed in haste, were scarcely on the ground when one of the most appalling storms I have ever witnessed, which left neither person nor baggage dry in any part. The sick were left on board the boat, and their number has much increased from the camp. The whole number of cases is fourteen; four deaths; no convalescents yet." The following day's report from Everett stated, "There have been eleven cases since my last, and three deaths. Three cases are, I think, convalescent." That same day Everett himself began showing the symptoms of the disease.[5]

By July 7, the third day of the outbreak on board the *Henry Clay*, Colonel Twiggs reported the death toll had reached four, with another eight men seriously ill. At this point, on the advice of Dr. Everett, Twigg landed his ship on the mainland approximately a mile south from Fort Gratiot on the St. Clair River. By the 9th the death toll on the *Henry Clay*

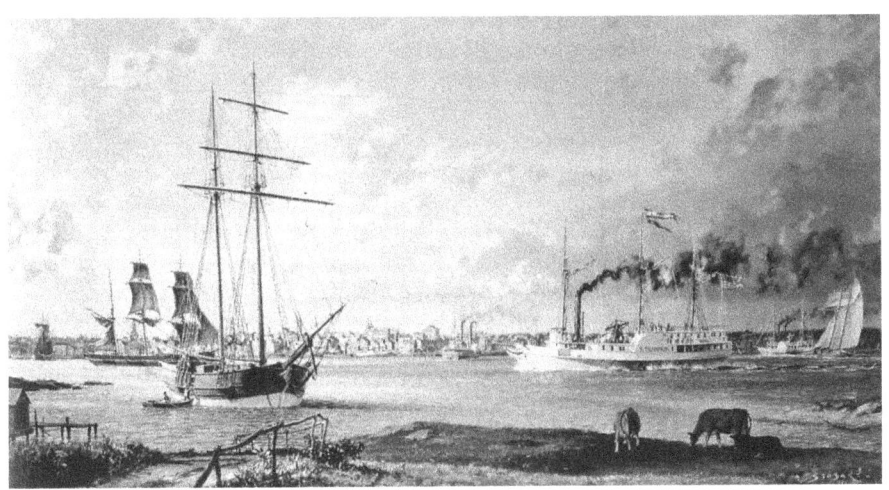

Steamship *Sheldon Thompson*, among those schooners that transported Scott and his troops (courtesy Burton Historical Collection, Detroit Public Library).

had reached 18. The dead included "the first officer who had been attacked, Lieutenant [Joseph] Clay, Fourth United States Infantry, and that Dr. Everett is now sick with cholera."[6] On July 16 Everett's death was reported.[7]

A graphic description of cholera was provided by an unnamed officer from his hospital bed at Fort Dearborn (Chicago) a week after the disease broke out among Scott's troops:

> We have got at last to our place of rendezvous, but in what a condition! We have travelled 600 miles [Buffalo to Chicago by way of Detroit] in a steam boat, crowded almost to suffocation, and the Asiatic cholera raging amongst us. The scenes on board the boat [the *Sheldon Thompson*, the only boat to arrive in Chicago by the 12th] are not to be described. Men died in six hours after being in perfect health. The steerage was crowded with the dying, and new cases were appearing on the deck, when the demon entered the cabin. The first case occurred at Fort Gratiot; the man attacked belonged to the company that I command. I found that the soldiers hesitated about attending him at first, so that I went to the sick man, felt his pulse and stood by his bed, and in a short time the soldiers became reconciled. This was only at first, for when the disease came upon us with fury, and the boat became a moving pestilence, every soldier who was well became a nurse for the sick. The disease was met with resolution, and never did a body of men stand more firmly by each other than the soldiers in our boat.
>
> To give you an idea of the disease; you remember Sergeant [Christian] Heyl: he was well at 9 o'clock in the morning — he was at the bottom of Lake Michigan, at 7 o'clock in the afternoon![8] I was officer of the day when we arrived, and had to remove all the sick men to the shore; I had scarcely got through my task, when I was thrown down on the deck almost as suddenly as if shot. As I was walking on the lower deck I felt my legs growing stiff from my knees downward. I went on the upper deck and walked violently to keep up a circulation of the blood. I felt suddenly a rush of blood from my feet upwards, and as it rose, my veins grew cold and my blood curdled. I was seized with a nausea at the stomach and a desire to vomit. My legs and hands were cramped with violent pain. The doctor gave me 8 grams of opium and made me rub my legs as fast as I could; he also made me drink a tumbler and a half full of raw brandy, and told me if I did not throw up the opium I would certainly be relieved, I did not throw it up and I was relieved, but not until I had had a violent spasm. The pain is excruciating. I am now out of danger.[9]

It is unclear exactly which treatment was employed on the soldier beyond the use of opium and brandy; he does not mention blood-letting, a common method of treatment at the time. Perhaps the best we can say is that

3. Cholera Among the Troops

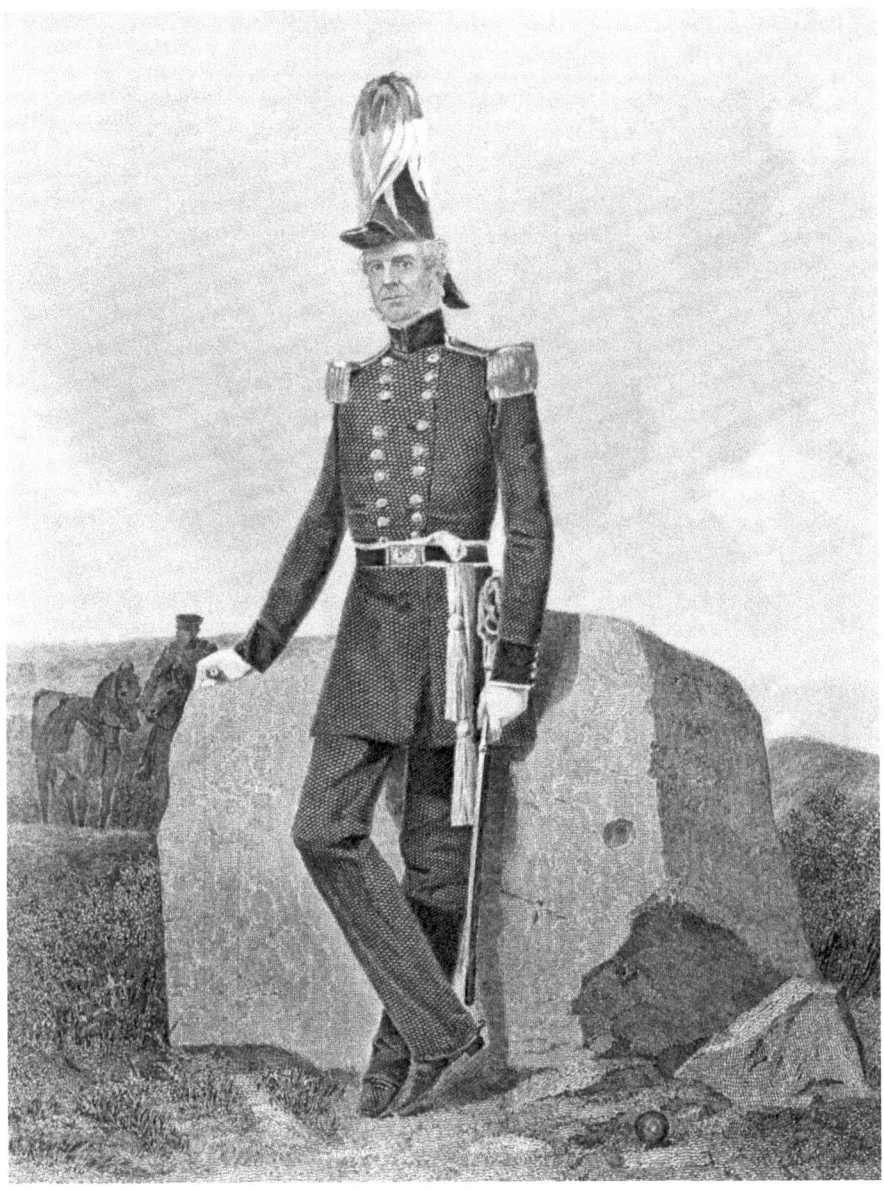

Colonel William Worth, aide and colleague of General Scott, who was among the latter's commanders in 1832. Worth died from cholera while serving in Texas during the 1849 outbreak. The city of Fort Worth was named in this honor (courtesy United States Military Academy).

given the options of treatments often used in dealing with cholera (see ch. 2), the doctors at least did no harm.

Scott's behavior during the initial period of the outbreak could only be considered as exemplary. Once the general realized the disease was present — at least on the *Henry Clay* — he transferred some of the (apparently) uninfected troops as well as the recent graduates of the United States Military Academy and himself to the *Sheldon Thompson*, which after initially docking at Detroit to take on needed provisions had pulled alongside the *Henry Clay*. The *Henry Clay* was by now docked at Hog Island. The transfer included approximately 50 troops under the command of Twiggs as well as Scott and his staff and other officers, including General North and Lieutenant-Colonel Alexander Cummings, a total of some 40 men.[10] But Scott was too late, and in fact it was unlikely that anything other than extreme quarantine measures would have made a difference anyway. The disease continued to break out, not only on the *Henry Clay* but on the other steamers as well. The one medical officer on the *Sheldon Thompson*, rather than maintaining a cool head in the face of a developing crisis, panicked. At that time cholera had not yet broken out on the ship. He proceeded to down a bottle of wine and took to his bunk.

Scott ordered the *Henry Clay* to continue past Detroit to Fort Gratiot while he took charge himself in dealing with the increasing number of cases that were now appearing. Scott's feelings towards the *Thompson's* surgeon were plain: "He ought to have died."[11] Scott was later commended in writing by Secretary of War Lewis Cass for his behavior in dealing with the illness among his men. Despite a scare later that fall, Scott never showed any evidence of developing the disease himself. Scott also ordered the members of the class of 1832 from the military academy to return to West Point. There are no reports that indicate any of those men contracted cholera.

Scott later commented upon his helplessness in the situation — facing an enemy he couldn't see while at the same time planning a military campaign: "He had never felt his entire helplessness and need of Divine Providence as he did upon the lakes in the midst of the Asiatic Cholera. Sentinels were of no use in warning of the enemy's approach. He could not storm his works, fortify against him, nor cut his way out, nor make terms of capitulation. There was no respect for a flag of truce, and his men were falling upon all sides from an enemy in his very midst."[12]

3. Cholera Among the Troops

The *Sheldon Thompson* meanwhile had remained free from cholera. On July 6 the steamer proceeded north towards Fort Mackinac, located on what is now Mackinac Island on the Straits of Mackinac, connecting Lake Huron with Lake Michigan. By the time the ship reached Mackinac Island on the 7th, four cases of cholera had appeared among the troops. All were hospitalized at the fort and all four subsequently succumbed to the disease. Since the outbreak on the ship appeared to be limited to the aforementioned four, the ship proceeded south in Lake Michigan towards Fort Dearborn. However, during the voyage an additional 21 cases developed by the 8th, and by the time the ship reached its destination on the 10th a total of 76 cases had developed, with 19 deaths among those infected.[13]

General Scott recognized the danger of troops infected with cholera possibly transmitting the disease to the garrison at Fort Dearborn. Scott ordered the as-yet-uninfected men to leave the fort and encamp some two miles away. Meanwhile the fort itself was converted into a hospital. The evacuation proved insufficient, as some infected troops had visited the nearby village of Chicago, spreading the infection there, while at the same time several of the garrison encamped outside the fort ignored orders and became infected as a result of returning to the fort. The epidemic did not subside until the end of July, at which point the army was able to resume its attempts to suppress the native uprising.

4

Detroit, Vintage 1832

To understand the cholera outbreaks in Detroit during the period between 1832 and later in that century, it is helpful to observe the evolution of what was originally a settlement, but which grew into a small city by the 1820s. In addition, a brief history of the origins of the settlement provides some perspective on later developments. As was the situation with many of the towns or villages established in what would someday become the midwestern United States, geography and resources were major factors in settlers moving to the territory of Michigan, as well as in laying out the plans for the original village of Detroit.

Michigan's geography can be attributed to mass glacial movements. As the glaciers retreated northward at the end of the Ice Age some twelve or more thousand years ago, the mantle underneath the ground surface was broken apart, causing a spread of clay, sand and gravel. At the same time, crystalline and sedimentary rocks degraded the glaciers and led to the deposition of ice. As a result, the soil in Michigan is newer, subject to greater aeration, and more pristine than soil in surrounding regions. Many minerals compose the glacial soil of Michigan. With this fresh land exposed, plants were able to thrive. Nutrients were plentiful, especially when the soil is compared with that in nearby regions. For instance, the phosphorus levels in southern Michigan soil were four times greater than levels measured in the soil of Illinois.[1]

In addition to healthy soil, southeast Michigan had a generous supply of fresh water. The majority of the land comprising today's Metro-Detroit region was flat, and as a result there was little drainage of water. Shallow ponds and swamps covered most of the land for at least a third of the year. This created a significant mosquito problem for the settlers. Since mosquitoes were able to breed in the stagnant pools of water that seemed to be everywhere, mosquito-borne diseases such as malaria became very common among the early settlers. In time, the settlers cleared the forests and carved out drainage systems, alleviating some of the problems as excess rain water or swamp water could be redirected.

Geographically, the Detroit River was the major means of travel for southeast Michigan's first settlers. Entering the river from nearby Lake Erie, the traveler could follow the coast of the territory until the river emptied into present-day Lake St. Clair, a distance of 32 miles. The northern portion of Lake St. Clair is linked with Lake Huron by the 40-mile-long St. Clair River. From Lake Huron the traveler could proceed north through the Straits of Mackinac, entering Lake Superior. Continuing west into Lake Michigan and proceeding south from that point, the traveler would circle the lower Michigan peninsula and arrive at Fort Dearborn and the nearby settlement of Chicago. This was the route Winfield Scott and his troops took as they traveled south from Buffalo, which is located on the eastern portion of Lake Erie, up the Detroit River to Detroit and Fort Gratiot, and subsequently to Fort Dearborn. Prior to Michigan's statehood in 1837, what is now the western portion of Michigan's Upper Peninsula was then part of Wisconsin Territory.

The use of the Detroit River was considered so vital to the settlement of the Michigan Territory that Congress on December 31, 1819, declared it to be a public highway.[2] The river is three miles across at its widest point and approximately one-half mile at its narrowest point at Detroit. The river depth varies from 10 to 60 feet, with an average of 34 feet, sufficient for passage of ships of significant size. Due to the flow of water between the Great Lakes, the Detroit River receives its supply from lakes Superior, Michigan and Huron. In addition, smaller sources of water and access include Lake St. Clair, Saginaw Bay, Green Bay and the thousands of streams that feed into the river. During the winter the Detroit River often freezes; the ice cover can be between 12 and 20 inches thick. Water levels are lowest during February and March, and highest during the summer months. There are 21 islands in the Detroit River with a combined shoreline of 72 miles, 33 of which are now portions of Canadian territory. The largest island, Grosse Isle, is approximately 10 square miles. As we have seen earlier, Hog Island — Belle Isle — played a role in determining where Scott's troops encamped once cholera had broken out on the steamboats.

Before European settlers arrived in Michigan, the state had an estimated 15,000 Native Americans, the major tribes being the Chippewa,

Ottawa, Potawatomi and Hurons. The first Europeans to visit Michigan were led by Commander Antoine de la Mothe Cadillac, reaching shore in present-day downtown Detroit in June 1701. Cadillac was accompanied by his nine-year-old son, his second-in-command Alphonse de Tonti, two priests and approximately 100 soldiers and workmen. They were traveling with Algonquin natives from Montreal with the intention of creating a permanent French settlement at the site and securing trade routes along the river and interior regions of the territory.

On July 23 Cadillac decided upon the present-day site of Detroit to build a settlement, the area being adjacent to the one of the narrowest widths of the Detroit River. The following day they began to build the fort, which they named Pontchartrain de Detroit (Straits of Pontchartrain) in honor of Cadillac's benefactor, Louis Phelypeaux, count of Pontchartrain, French chancellor and controller-general of finances; the site was renamed Fort du Detroit in 1751. By winter, Cadillac and his men had built log houses and developed Native American settlements around Fort Pontchartrain for protection and trade; these settlements were inhabited by members of the local tribes.

The early 1700s were a time of exploration and expansion of the fort. At the same time relations with the local native tribes were not always peaceful. In February 1704 Cadillac recorded that there were nearly 2,000 Native Americans encamped near the fort, seemingly in good spirits and on friendly terms with the French. However, on June 6, 1706, an argument between Miami and Ottawa tribesmen broke out when one of the fort's priests was kidnapped; the priest was eventually killed. In retaliation the soldiers murdered 30 Ottawa natives. The following year a council of native chiefs met at the fort, with Cadillac leading the discussions in an attempt to address the problems between the new settlers and local natives. Cadillac's men began to settle in the area surrounding the fort, with the establishment of "ribbon farms" that began at the river and in narrow strips extended inland. Some present-day extensions of streets near the downtown area still reflect some of the layout originated by the French at the time of Cadillac.

French settlers continued to settle in the region, a situation that only exacerbated troubles with the local native peoples; by the 1740s the population had increased to more than 900 persons. In 1747 soldiers were sent from Montreal to the fort to help defend against attacks by

4. Detroit, Vintage 1832

the Native Americans. By this time relations between France and England were deteriorating, and many of these attacks were the result of encouragement by the English. The situation came to a head during what became known in North America as the French and Indian War. Detroit played a critical role during the fighting as both French and English soldiers arrived in the region. In 1760 the fort was surrendered to the British and remained in British control until after the Revolutionary War.

With the end of the war in 1763, Detroit continued to grow and thrive as a trading post. The population increased to more than 2,000 by the time of the American revolution. The region remained in British hands during the war, but with independence achieved, the 1783 Treaty of Paris resulted in Detroit being returned to the United States as a portion of the Northwest Territory; Colonel John Frederick Hamtramck officially declared Detroit to be part of the United States in 1796.

By the end of the eighteenth century Detroit had become a highly successful commercial center. Still largely a fort, the site boasted a wharf, citadel, shops, taverns and some 300 houses, all situated close to each other in the region now bounded by Griswold, Cass and Larned streets. The legislature of the Northwest Territory incorporated Detroit as a town by an act that took effect in February 1802. Following a devastating fire in 1805, apparently started when a cigar was lit in the stable attached to John Harvey's bakery near the center of town, and which burned much of the settlement,[3] Judge Augustus Woodward developed plans for the rebuilding of the town. Woodward's idea was that streets would radiate outward, analogous to the spokes on a wheel. At the time the boundaries of the area reached what is now Grand Circus Park, bounded by Adams Avenue in Woodward's plan. The area was rapidly revitalized, and in September 1806 Detroit was officially incorporated as a city by the territorial legislature. Solomon Sibley was appointed by the territorial governor as the first mayor. Early in that decade Father Gabriel Richard, a French Roman-Catholic priest, came to Detroit to serve as assistant pastor at St. Anne's Church. Founded in 1701 by Cadillac, St. Anne's is still the second-oldest continuously operating parish in the country. The first school opened by Richard burned in the 1805 fire, so Richard continued his work by ministering to the Native Americans in the region.

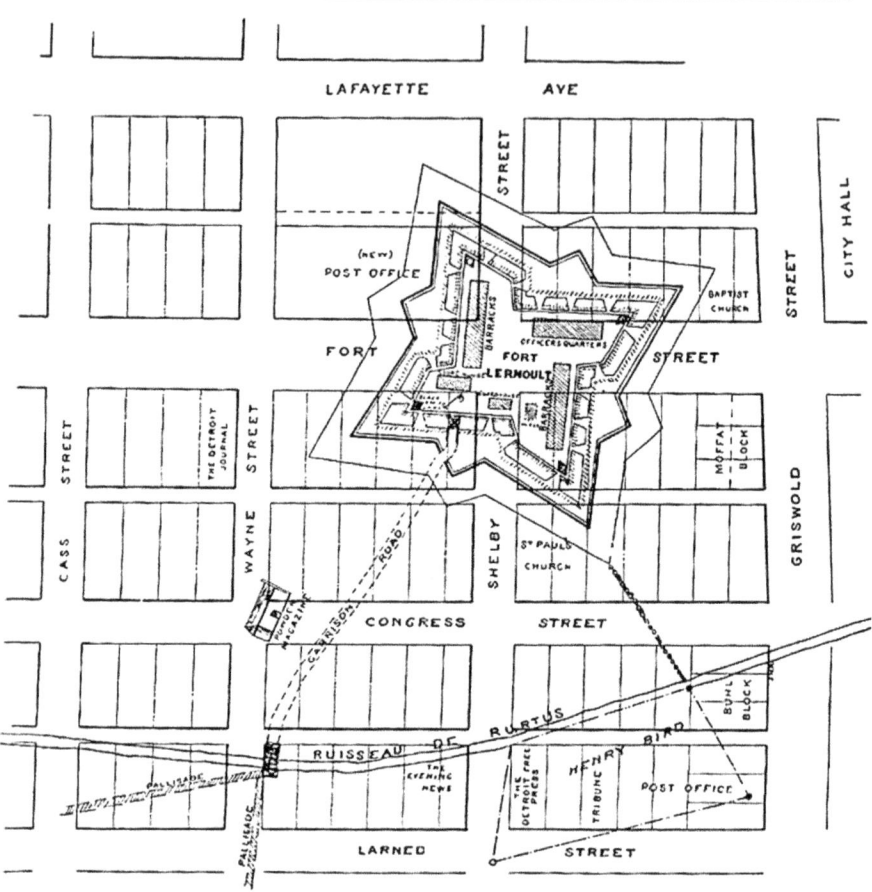

Fort Lernoult vs. Detroit City Plan (ca. 1800s) (Burton, 1922). Later renamed Fort Shelby, the fort was surrendered to the British during the War of 1812.

During the War of 1812, Fort Shelby, built within the city as the site of the garrison, was surrendered to the British, as described earlier. Once the city was returned to the United States in 1815 the population continued to increase. Several factors contributed to this increase, most notably the completion of the Erie Canal, which reduced travel time between New York City and Detroit from several months to less than a week. An additional feature that improved convenience for westward travel was the completion of a highway between Detroit and Chicago (roughly the path of Michigan Route 12 today). Numerous settlers also

4. Detroit, Vintage 1832

passed through Detroit, and supplying these travelers with needed supplies and equipment became one of the early growth industries of the city. To encourage western settlement, Congress passed a land act in 1820 that allowed settlers to purchase land cheaply, for $1.25 an acre, with a minimum purchase of 80 acres. As these settlers moved west from Detroit they often set down roots wherever they found fertile land — plentiful in the territory — and where they found streams for the construction of waterwheels. Many of the current suburbs of Detroit — Oak Park, Royal Oak, Plymouth — originated in this manner.

The passage of so many travelers through the city not surprisingly overwhelmed the sanitation needs of the population. The Detroit River became a dumping ground for garbage and waste, reaching a level so intolerable that in 1820 the city government levied a tax for the purpose of clearing the river.

The governing body of the city also underwent a change during this period. In 1824 the territorial legislature created the Common Council, consisting of five aldermen, the mayor and a recorder, as the governing body for Detroit; the number of aldermen was increased to seven in 1827. That same year, 1827, the city began the installation of its first water system, eliminating the need for the citizenry to acquire water by collecting it directly from the river. The system included two horse-driven pumps on the wharf, which sent the water to the top of a pump house. The water then flowed to a 9,500 gallon reservoir, located on what today is the corner of Jefferson and Randolph streets, from which water was distributed through a series of water mains. That same year Congress approved a request to develop a series of roads linking Detroit with Chicago (including State Route 12) and Detroit with Fort Gratiot (present-day Port Huron).

Waves of Irish immigrants began arriving in Detroit by 1830, many settling in the area subsequently labeled the Corktown District — later the site of professional baseball for more than 100 years. A large influx of German settlers also began settling during this same period so that by the time of the 1832 cholera outbreak, the population of the town had reached 4,500 persons, with the surrounding Wayne County, including Detroit and at the time much of eastern Michigan, incorporating a population of nearly 24,000 persons.

Evolution of the Detroit Water and Sanitation Systems

The Detroit River served as the primary source of water until a direct public water system was developed early in the nineteenth century. Residents of the settlement simply went to the river with buckets, which they dipped into the water, and carried them back to their homes. Since fire was always a hazard in the wooden log or frame homes, citizens of the town were required to maintain a ready supply of water on premises. Horse-drawn carts carrying vessels of water could deliver their supplies to those homes whose residents were unable to collect their own water.

The problem of sewage was easily addressed in the manner of the time. Wastewater simply flowed along open sewers into the river, the same river that supplied household water. While residents might be willing to tolerate the smells, at least up to a point, the concept of waterborne diseases had to wait several generations.

The 1805 fire changed much of the way with which the settlement dealt with the water problem. A series of public wells with attached pumps was developed, but proved inadequate as a permanent solution. In 1824 Lewis Cass, the Michigan territorial governor, and the Legislative Council authorized Peter Berthelet from Montreal to construct the aforementioned wharf and pump at the foot of Randolph Street, now the site of the entrance to the Detroit-Windsor (Canada) tunnel. The construction was paid for with a small tax levied

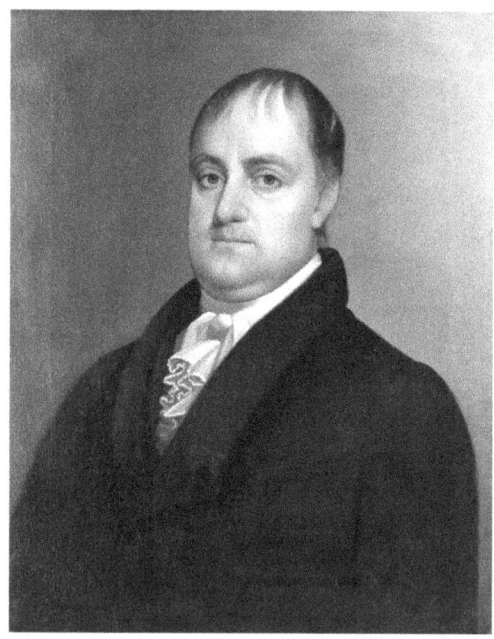

Lewis Cass, territorial governor of Michigan, 1813–1831 (courtesy Burton Historical Collection, Detroit Public Library).

4. Detroit, Vintage 1832

on the citizens, and Berthelet received a 99-year lease.[4] The terms by which Berthelet was authorized provided that "all persons who may reside within the city of Detroit, shall at all times be free of wharfage or other expenses, entitled to take and draw water for their use and convenience, and for that purpose a free use of said wharf shall be given, for carts, wagons, sleighs, or other machinery, and be used in drawing and carrying away the water."[5]

In 1825 the Detroit Common Council granted Bethuel Farrand authority to supply water for Detroit. Farrand transferred the authority to pump-maker Rufus Wells a year later, and by the end of 1827 the system was supplying water to the city; it remained functional until 1850.[6] The water bill for families was fixed at $10 per year. The system quickly proved inadequate for the size of the population, and despite the sale of bonds with the purpose of upgrading the system, the citizens of Detroit still obtained much of their water directly from the Detroit River.

In 1829 Wells organized his business's charter into a new company, the Hydraulic Company, which attempted to supplement its supply of water by drilling for groundwater. The first attempts were carried out near the site of Fort and Shelby streets. Despite drilling as deep as 260 feet, the operation proved unable to locate the groundwater and the venture was abandoned.[7] Instead, a new reservoir was built on the site where the drilling operation had come to naught, one with a storage capacity of some 22,000 gallons. Water mains consisted of hollowed-out logs, with the individual units linked with sleeves of lead.[8] An even larger reservoir, holding nearly 120,000 gallons, was built in 1831. The first reservoir using iron pipes, replacing those made from hollowed-out logs, was started in 1837 along Jefferson Avenue between Randolph Street and Woodward Avenue.

The growing population in the city created more problems than the need for sufficient drinking water. Outhouses—"privies"—remained the primary means of household elimination of bodily wastes. Open cesspools not only created unpleasant odors, they were a breeding ground for any water-borne disease introduced into the city. Untreated sewage simply washed into the river. While intake pipes were supposedly placed towards the center of the river, away from the raw sewage that accumulated along the shoreline, the water supply could not help but become contaminated. The relatively small width of the river at that site, less than a mile, only exacerbated the problem. The Common Council was given the authorization to construct a sewer system by an act in April 1824. Concern was expressed, however, as to whether the construction of such a system would actually be detrimental to the public health. The reasoning was perhaps convoluted, and given the passage of time it is hard to understand the question behind any delay. The most reasonable explanation for the lack of progress on the issue was the prevailing belief that disease was a function of miasmas or odors that would emanate from the sewer were it to be constructed, and not necessarily the sewage per se. Despite the authorization of $50,000 in bonds for the development of a functioning sewer system, nothing was accomplished on a permanent basis until several years after the 1832 cholera outbreak.

The first attempt in the construction of an actual sewer system took place in 1827 when the Common Council adopted the following: "Resolved, that the drain or ravine commonly called the River Savoyard, be deepened from the outlet into the Detroit River, through the farm of Governor [Lewis] Cass, to the line of the military reservation, with the consent of the proprietor of said farm; and that a drain in continuation thereof be extended through the said reservation in the alley between Congress and Larned Streets to its easterly termination."[9] Construction began on what would be an open sewer, with the walls constructed of timbers that originally had been part of Fort Shelby. The sewer followed the same path as had the original creek, and was utilized as a means to dispose of city sewage until the larger system was built several years later.

The first functioning sewage system actually constructed in Detroit, the Grand Sewer, was authorized in 1836 and built of stone and brick at a cost of some $23,000. The sewer enclosed Savoyard Creek (River Savoyard above), which flowed from present-day Cadillac Square to the foot of Third Street where it dumped — literally — the untreated sewage into the Detroit River and which had been designed by the Common Council several years earlier as an open sewer. The Savoyard Creek in its more pristine days had been a ready source of fresh fish. Originally called by the French Ruissau des Hurons (brook or creek of the Hurons), after the name of the tribe which was located nearby on the Detroit River, the creek originated in the marsh then found at the corner of Brush and Congress streets, near the present-day Wayne County Building. The creek originally meandered westward through a meadow, largely following the route of Congress Street through the current business area of downtown Detroit, and turned south near today's Joe Louis Arena. Eventually, however, the population began using the creek as a convenient open sewer. In 1827 the Common Council had converted the creek into a sewer as described above. By the time it was converted into part of the sewage system during the 1830s, the stench had become so offensive that the population was happy to see it covered. The site is now occupied by the Buhl Building on Congress and Griswold streets. The route of the original creek may also be seen in the depression in the street south of the corner of Fort and Griswold.[10]

Origins of the Detroit Health Department

Meanwhile it was during this period that Detroit began to deal with other aspects of urban life that were directly affected by water and sanitation issues, including public health. The earliest known recorded references by the Common Council to concerns affecting the public health were in 1825 when recommendations were made in dealing with public "nuisances," standing bodies of sewage water. The population of Detroit that year was recorded in the *Gazette* as 1,325, not including the garrison within the city or the nearly 500 persons living outside the city limits, a significant population.[11] What were the specific nuisances with which the council had to deal? A report recorded in the minutes of March 12, 1827, described some dozen of the most important, two of which dealt with issues of public health: "the removal of disease breeding refuse from the margin of the river," and construction of the sewer as described above.[12] That year the Common Council also appointed a committee of three physicians, the purpose of which was to provide for the council recommendations of "such measures both general and particular embracing objects both of public and individual police as they may consider conducive to the health of the city."[13]

The first reference to a formal Detroit board of health was recorded by the Common Council in August 1831. The board initially consisted of two physicians: Dr. John Leffingwell Whiting and Dr. Randall S. Rice. Both Whiting and Rice were also serving as assistant engineers with the Detroit fire department. Whiting was also vice-president and Rice the secretary of the Medical Society of the Territory of Michigan. An interesting sidelight is that on January 8, 1828, at a meeting of the society, Rice read into the minutes a letter from army physician Dr. William Beaumont, dated August 1827, in which Beaumont described "experiments on the digestive powers of the stomach." Beaumont inserted undigested meat into a stomach wound of a patient being treated near the fort on Mackinac Island and observed the digestive process. The experiment is now considered a classic study; the building in which the experiment took place in 1822 is still present on the island.[14] In October the council expressed concern because "there is reason to apprehend the arrival at this port of a vessel or vessels on board of which there may be cases of smallpox." The concern may have been warranted as a report from the Board of Health referred to "a black man — labouring under unequivocal confluent smallpox."[15] Whiting and Rice, the health officers who had been appointed to determine whether any travelers or crew members on incoming ships represented a threat to the city's public health, were able to set the minds of the aldermen at ease:

> The undersigned, Health officers for the City of Detroit, have, in pursuance of instructions from the Common Council, made diligent inquiries, and have ascertained that no contagious disease exists at the present time in the city. Since the last report a schooner called the *United States* has arrived from Green Bay in which were two persons who had the smallpox [perhaps including the individual mentioned above]. But she was not allowed to come to the wharves and has this morning sailed for Buffalo. [In effect the smallpox became Buffalo's problem.]

They would further add, "The most vigorous measures have been adopted, and are now in process, to vaccinate all persons liable to the contagion of the smallpox, and to prevent the communication of that disease."[16] Presumably, health officers went through the city ensuring that susceptible persons had been vaccinated, no small task, as citizens were often suspicious of the vaccination process, a challenge faced by the medical profession even during the present day. Skepticism of the vaccination process may better be understood in the context of the period. The vaccine often consisted of fresh lymphatic fluid from a lesion of cowpox on the udder of a calf or cow. If any contamination of the vaccination material occurred, the recipient could very well develop a life-threatening infection.

4. Detroit, Vintage 1832

The following year, 1832, the board was expanded with the addition of Dr. (Marvin?) Henry and Dr. Marshall Chapin.[17] During the two outbreaks of cholera which took place during the 1830s, the seven aldermen on the Common Council aldermen were temporarily added to the board as well.[18]

The vocation of physician was an honorable one, critical to the health of the individual as well as that of the city itself. In the 1830s, of course, with only a rudimentary knowledge of the basis of contagious disease and few effective methods of treatment, a physician could do little more than provide moral support to the afflicted individual or the family. Even so, such support could still provide a measure of solace:

> When age has impaired the organs of life, and man must die, when all the balm of Gilead has no power to preserve the system from decay; when complicated diseases fasten upon the vitals and frame of middle age, youth or childhood, of such fierce and conflicting tendencies, that the power of medicine is set at defiance, and nature must be left alone in the fatal struggle — then comes the physician's gloomy hour. He must hear groans that he cannot alleviate, and he must witness the breaking up of those earthly ties which are among the bitter pangs of death.
>
> Yet under all circumstances, how welcome are the visits of the physician! He comes with an educated mind, and pleasing manners to cheer scenes which the gay world have withdrawn from, and where even friendship is slow to enter.[19]

As effective as Rice and Whiting may have been in sparing Detroit from an epidemic of smallpox, they were unprepared for the events that would take place several months later. Noble sentiments reflecting the importance of the city's physicians would be put to the test as they discovered there was little that could be done to prevent the outbreak of cholera. The conditions necessary for the epidemic — an impure water supply obtained from the nearby river, and a rudimentary sanitation system that could not help but release contaminated sewage into the river — were in place.

5

Detroit, Cholera and the Black Hawk War: Events of 1832

> If he [political rival Lewis Cass] saw any live, fighting Indians it was more than I did, but I had a good many bloody struggles with the mosquitoes.—Abraham Lincoln[1]

The epidemic of cholera in Detroit in 1832 arose as the product of violent hostilities between the Native American tribes and the local militia in Illinois and Indiana in what has been termed the Black Hawk War. In a later time the victims of the outbreak might have been referred to as collateral damage. Earlier chapters have described the exposure to cholera of troops under the command of General Scott, either in Buffalo or several days earlier in New York City while on their way to participate in suppressing the uprising. Those troops subsequently became the source for the outbreak in Detroit that July.

The Black Hawk War

The Black Hawk War is one of the lesser known conflicts in American history. There were relatively few battlefield casualties on the American side of the conflict; Native American casualties numbered many hundreds. Black Hawk himself was captured and subsequently brought to Washington where he met with President Andrew Jackson.

So what was the Black Hawk War, and with the local militia on scene, what was President Jackson' purpose in ordering troops from Virginia to participate in the conflict? It was this decision by the president that proved the harbinger of Detroit's first great cholera epidemic.

5. Detroit, Cholera and the Black Hawk War

The Black Hawk War had its origins in 1804, when the Treaty of St. Louis was signed. This was one of 13 treaties established between Governor William Henry Harrison of the newly established Indiana Territory (including present-day Illinois) and the Sauk and Meskwaki (Fox) as well as other tribes. The Native Americans signed over much of the land in western Illinois and Indiana to the United States. As a result the natives were forced west of the Mississippi River. Among the native leaders less than pleased with the arrangement was Black Sparrow Hawk, generally referred to as Black Hawk by the white settlers. The deep resentment these treaties engendered among the native populations was one of many reasons they sided with the British against the Americans during the War of 1812.

In the years following the Treaty of Ghent, which ended that war in 1815, white settlers began pouring into region, encroaching on lands that had served as ancestral homes for the natives over many generations. A single example may illustrate the attitude of the white settlers towards the native tribes. In 1830 a band of natives, known as the British Band for their continued friendly relations with the British garrison at Malden in northern Indiana, discovered upon their return from a hunt that white settlers had destroyed their lodges and fields. The whites even desecrated the graves of their ancestors. In May 1831, Black Hawk responded by informing the settlers along the Rock River, a tributary of the Mississippi in northern Illinois, that he was planning on reclaiming the land, some of which had been the site of his birthplace and youth. Between 400 and 600 Native American warriors made the threat credible. In response, the frightened settlers called on the recently elected governor, John Reynolds (1788–1865), for military help. Reynolds called out 1,600 men from the state militia as well as ten companies of regulars under the command of General Edmund Gaines (1777–1849). Gaines, a veteran of the War of 1812 and the Seminole Wars, which several years later followed that conflict, was only too happy to participate: "It is my duty to state to you that I have ordered six companies of the regular troops stationed at Jefferson Barracks [St. Louis] to embark tomorrow morning and to repair forthwith to the spot occupied by the hostile Sacs. To this detachment I shall, if necessary, add four companies. With this force I am satisfied I shall be able to repel the invasion and give security to the frontier inhabitants of the state."[2]

The military response by Reynolds and Gaines proved sufficient to force Black Hawk back across the Mississippi. On the 30th of June that year (1831), a treaty was signed between Reynolds and Gaines and

> the Chiefs and Braves of the band of Sac Indians—usually called the "British Band" of Rock River—with their old allies of the Pottawatamie, Winnebagoe and Kickapoo Nations ... that the British band of Sac Indians are required peaceably to submit to the authority of the friendly chiefs and braves of the united Sac and Fox nation, and at all times hereafter to reside and hunt with them upon their own lands, *west of the Mississippi River* [italics added] ... and no one of the said band shall ever be permitted to recross said river to the place of their usual residence ... without the express permission of the President of the United States or the Governor of the State of Illinois.[3]

And what did the natives receive in return? The United States guaranteed "to the united Sac and Fox nations, including the said 'British Band' of Sac Indians, the integrity of all the lands claimed by them westward of the Mississippi River, pursuant to the treaties of the years 1825 and 1830." Black Hawk, along with 27 chiefs and warriors, had no choice but to sign the treaty.[4] The agreement was broken, however, the first week of April 1832 when Black Hawk, accompanied by 500 Fox and Kickapoo warriors and their families, some 1,500 in all, crossed the Mississippi again in hopes of regaining his land. It is likely Black Hawk was influenced by a Winnebagoe native known as the prophet, who convinced Black Hawk that he would be joined in an alliance with other tribes in sufficient numbers to defeat any military force which opposed him. On the 16th of April Governor Reynolds again called upon the militia to assemble. In response to Reynold's call some 1,600 men gathered and marched to nearby Fort Armstrong, near Rock Island.[5]

General Henry Atkinson was the commander of the Fort Armstrong garrison. The militia raised by Reynolds were temporarily mustered into the army, and with 400–500 of Atkinson's regulars began a march on May 9 to the Rock River, where Black Hawk and his warriors were to be found. Two battalions under the command of Major Isaiah Stillman and Major David Bailey were ordered to reconnoiter Black Hawk's encampment. Discovering the nearby presence of the Americans, Black Hawk sent several emissaries with a flag of parley to negotiate some sort of truce. The militia, however, consisted largely of untrained and undisciplined troops, and through a series of miscalculations several of Black Hawk's emissaries were killed. The Americans continued in pursuit of the remaining emissaries, stumbled into an ambush laid by Black Hawk, and panicked and fled. The skirmish became known as the Battle of Stillman's Run, though it is unclear whether Stillman himself was present. One detachment of militia under the command of Captain John Adams attempted to make a stand, but they were overrun and lost all 12 men.[6] The small nearby creek was subsequently named Stillman's Run. Abraham Lincoln may have been one of the members of the Illinois militia who helped bury Adams' men.[7]

Following the skirmish Black Hawk and his men withdrew into what would later become southern Wisconsin. The Illinois militia refused to follow — a common problem when dealing with state militia and their reluctance to pass state boundaries — and despite a call by Governor Reynolds for additional militia to be mustered in for the duration, Black Hawk was able to escape. Questions were raised as to whether Atkinson, who had never been the commander of as large a force as was under his direction, was even sufficiently competent to continue the war against Black Hawk. Doubts concerning Atkinson's abilities soon reached the office of the president, who even before the news about the fighting at Stillman's Run had reach him, had informed representatives from Illinois about his concerns "that General Jackson, then president of the United States, had stated that he had furnished adequate means for prosecuting the war against the Sacs and Foxes and had placed General Atkinson in command, and that if he, General Atkinson, did not terminate the war in thirty days, he would dismiss him from the army."[8]

Perhaps recognizing the inadequacies of General Atkinson as well as those of the local militia, Reynolds made a request to the federal government for more troops — specifically regular army — to help in suppressing of the uprising, and in response President Andrew Jackson ordered General Scott and a thousand regulars to travel from Virginia west to Illinois. As recounted earlier, it was during the travel through New York that these troops were exposed to the cholera outbreak. Scott was an obvious choice for commanding the American troops and militia. At 6'5" and 200-plus pounds, his imposing figure was the epitome of an army officer. The military tactics and bravery he had exhibited during the War of 1812 had made him a national hero. Scott (1786–1866) would spend much of his long life in the military before retiring in the early days of the Civil War. And in trying to bring a measure of discipline to the settlers and backwoodsmen who constituted the militia, there was probably no better choice than Scott. The only real hesitation on the part of Jackson in making the decision was due to the political ambitions and political allies of Scott. But that can wait.

Scott and his men arrived at Fort Dearborn on July 10. During the 11-day journey from Virginia the troops had been exposed to cholera, either while traveling through New York City or during their time in Buffalo, and, it was during the passage from Buffalo to Detroit that the disease appeared among Scott's men. After spending two weeks with his troops as the cholera outbreak finally subsided — more than 50 men died and another 80 barely managed to survive by the time he reached the fort — Scott and a small escort on the 29th of July traveled towards Prairie du Chien in northern Illinois; Colonel Abraham Eustis followed with the bulk of the troops. Upon arrival Scott was to replace General Atkinson as commander of the force.

However, as events played out, Scott never actually assumed command in the subsequent fighting. Troops still under the command of General Atkinson now pursued Black Hawk across the state line into Michigan Territory,[9] finally cornering the Indians in what became known as the Battle of Wisconsin Heights, located near what is now Sauk City, Wisconsin. On July 21 some 700 men commanded by Colonel Henry Dodge occupied a ridge overlooking the river, and when Black Hawk and his warriors attempted to cross, Dodge and his men began firing; a bayonet charge by the Americans ended the battle. When night approached Black Hawk withdrew from the field. Approximately 70 of Black Hawk's men were killed, with more wounded. The Americans suffered only one death, with eight others wounded. Following the battle some of the noncombatants among the Sac and Fox — old men, women and children — also attempted to cross the river but were fired upon by some of the regular army troops; approximately 15 men and 32 women and children were killed in what was considered a massacre.[10]

Atkinson and his force, now consisting of 400 regular army troops and 1,300 militia, continued their pursuit of Black Hawk. The Native Americans were now reduced to a near starving condition. On August 1 in what was known as the Battle of Bad Axe, located near present-day Victory, Wisconsin, the Americans trapped Black Hawk's band on the east bank of the Mississippi. Following two days of fighting Black Hawk

5. Detroit, Cholera and the Black Hawk War

attempted to surrender. As a monument marking the site of the battle is inscribed, "On the eve of August 1, 1832, Blackhawk and his men with a flag of truce, went to the head of this island to surrender to the captain of steamer *Warrior*. Whites on board asked, 'Are you Winnebagoes [American allies] or Sacs?' 'Sacs,' replied Black Hawk. A load of canister was at once fired, killing 28 Indians suing for peace." During the fighting approximately 150 Indians were killed, many of whom drowned. Seventeen of Atkinson's men died as well.

Black Hawk was not injured and did manage to escape. However, with his force nearly annihilated by now — of the 1,500 men, women and children who had originally crossed the Mississippi in May, fewer than 150 remained — soon afterwards Black Hawk himself surrendered at Prairie du Chien. The signing of the treaty had to be delayed as cholera broke out among both the settlers and natives. It may have been carried by members of Scott's force or members of the militia who had been exposed; the distance from Fort Dearborn to Fort Armstrong at Rock Island where the treaty was to be signed was only some 180 miles, and the disease could easily have spread from Fort Dearborn. While battle casualties among the soldiers had been relatively modest, approximately 500 men succumbed to cholera before the epidemic subsided. Ironically, few of Scott's men were ever engaged in battle and most never left the vicinity of Fort Dearborn or Chicago. Deaths were nearly entirely the result of disease.

The treaty was finally signed on September 15, marking the end of native occupation on the eastern bank of the Mississippi in that region. The remaining tribes, primarily Winnebagoe by now, "sold" their remaining lands in Illinois and Michigan Territory, and in return received land west of the Mississippi along with schools and subsidies.[11] Black Hawk was brought east as a prisoner, though allotted a surprising amount of freedom. In Washington, D.C., he met both President Jackson and Secretary of War Lewis Cass. After a few weeks of imprisonment in Fortress Monroe in Virginia, Black Hawk was released and began a return trip that took him through both eastern and western cities, including a brief stay in Detroit where he was housed in the Mansion House Hotel, then located at Jefferson Avenue and Cass Street. The receptions he received were not always kind, no surprise given the bitterness that remained in the aftermath of the war. Black Hawk finally re-crossed the Mississippi River, eventually settling in Iowa Territory where he died in 1838.

Events of the Black Hawk War Bring Cholera to Detroit: 1832

As described in the previous chapter, when Governor John Reynolds requested federal troops to aid in suppressing the Indian uprising, President Jackson authorized General Scott to lead the troops under his command to Fort Dearborn. The route took them through New York City and Buffalo, along the way exposing them to cholera, which had broken out in each city. On July 2 the steamers *Henry Clay* and *Sheldon Thompson* left Buffalo with a total of nine companies of infantry as well as two companies of infantry plus recruits. Scott was on the *Sheldon Thompson*. On the 4th an additional two steamers left Buffalo.

That same day, the 4th, cholera broke out on the *Henry Clay*. Whether the source had been exposure in one of the cities or on the ship itself cannot be determined with certainty; while the *Henry Clay* had been previously used to transport immigrants among whom the disease had broken out, it had been thoroughly cleaned with chloride of lime before transporting the troops. Disinfection of the vessel suggests some recognition of human passage of the disease. Regardless of the source of the outbreak, cholera had become a full-fledged epidemic on the ship by the time it reached Detroit.

As the *Henry Clay* approached Detroit it notified the city of its arrival by firing a cannon as it neared Sandwich Point across the river, now the site of the city of Windsor, Ontario. The vessel docked and allowed two passengers to leave the ship.[12] Whether or not these passengers had already been exposed to cholera is unknown. It is also unclear whether the men were actually passengers on the ship, or had been sent from Detroit to communicate with the captain as was reported in the local media:

SPASMODIC CHOLERA IN DETROIT.

We are obliged to announce to our readers that the Spasmodic Cholera has made its appearance in this city. As might be expected the prevalence of such a malignant disease among us, has produced very general alarm among our citizens.

The first case occurred on the 5th inst. among the troops on board the *Henry Clay*. The subject, who was a soldier of intemperate habits expired, after an illness of seven hours. Others were soon after taken ill, and all of them exhibited the usual symptoms which are said to attend the disease. The vessel was ordered to leave the port, and she proceeded to Hog Island where she was furnished with supplies from this city for her voyage to Chicago.

On Friday [July 6], two cases occurred in town. The individuals had been employed, the day previous, *to communicate with the boat* [italics added]. One of them recovered, the other died the next day. On Saturday and Sunday, other cases occurred. Monday, at 12:00, the Board of Health made a report, which stated that the whole number of cases which had occurred in the city up to that time, including the nine cases which had occurred at the Military Storehouse, amounted to 17; nine of whom died, 5 soldiers were numbered among the dead. The remaining were convalescent.[13]

Several facts are clear from the story as reported. Since cholera had already been reported on board, the ship was ordered to dock upriver on Hog Island. But the attempt at quarantine proved to be too late. Whether the contact between the *Henry Clay* and the city involved the debarkation of two passengers, or whether the two individuals sent to contact the ship were the actual sources, cholera appeared in Detroit shortly after the ship arrived. We also see an attempt to explain the first case that occurred on the ship, the victim being "a soldier of intemperate habits." In other words, the soldier was a drunk.

The attempt to associate the liberal use of "alcoholic beverages" with increased risk of contracting the disease, particularly among soldiers and the "lower classes" of society, was certainly not limited to Detroit. A story that originated in New York described the current cholera epidemic in that city as follows:

> We have already mentioned the remarkable fact that of 204 cholera patients admitted to the Park Hospital [New York City] down to a certain date, 198 were intemperate. We can now add, from the best authority, that of all the patients admitted to Corlaer's Hook Hospital,[14] down to the present time, four-fifths were intemperate; and that while, of the collapsed cases, only 35 percent of the temperate cases have died, 71 percent of the intemperate have died.... The whole number of persons carried off by cholera in this city since the 1st of July, according to there port of interments [sic], is 2295; of which number it is a low estimate to suppose that 1500 were decidedly intemperate.... A withdrawal of 1500 drunkards from our population, must have a very perceptible effect in the moral purification of the city.[15]

It would not be hard to interpret the writer's prejudice to read that the victims had only themselves to blame, topped with a "good riddance."

The *Sheldon Thompson* and General Scott arrived shortly afterwards, and with so many cases of cholera appearing on the *Henry Clay*, the general ordered both steamers to proceed to Fort Gratiot, where the sick could receive better care. Once the passengers reached the shore, over 150 of the soldiers deserted in panic, and in attempting to spare themselves exposure to the disease fled downriver into the wilderness. Many of them died along the way, failing to reach whatever destination they had hoped to reach. Some may have died from exposure or hunger, others perhaps from cholera itself. Even weeks later travelers along the roads reported seeing dead men, some partially eaten by wild animals.[16] The report on the incident subsequently filed by General Scott confirmed the events described in the *Democratic Free Press*:

> When I landed here [Fort Gratiot] I had with me four companies of the finest looking recruits I have seen for many years. The panic is so great among them that the desertions have reduced the number to sixty-eight [from the original number of greater than 200]. It is reported that many of them (deserters) are dying on the roads. On the same date General Twiggs reports that he had ordered sixteen cadets, who were with his command, to leave camp and to report at West Point on the 1st of September next; thus affording an opportunity to these gentlemen of spending nearly two months at their home.[17]

The bodies of the deserters who died in the wilderness were later gathered up and buried in the cemetery at Fort Gratiot. One of the dead reportedly had been the son of Kentucky senator Henry Clay. Clay did indeed lose a son, who was killed during the Mexican War 16 years later. But the report of the loss of a son at Fort Gratiot was in error.[18] Survivors were occasionally observed, marching towards some unknown destination. Likely due to the fear of contracting the same disease, few of the living they encountered would be willing to provide them with food or water.

A particularly vivid account was provided nearly three decades later by another eyewitness to the events that July: Augustus Walker, captain of the *Sheldon Thompson*, in response to an inquiry by the *Chicago Tribune*. Walker's account encompasses the description of events at Fort Gratiot as well as subsequent events as his ship continued on the lakes towards their destination, Fort Dearborn (Chicago). In addition to corroborating the description of events as recounted earlier by an officer (chapter 3), Walker provided perspective from his role as the ship's captain.

5. Detroit, Cholera and the Black Hawk War

It is interesting at this late date, after the lapse of more than a quarter century, to review the past and glean therefrom statistics and data, which, though small in themselves, are nevertheless important as they serve as connecting links in the chain of events which have a direct bearing on the extensive commerce of our lakes, as well as the increasing growth and the rapid development of the resources of wealth in your city and State, which have hardly a parallel in history.

It will be borne in mind that at that time few traces of civilization could be seen, after passing the Straits of Mackinaw [dividing the upper and lower peninsulas of Michigan]; nothing like lighthouses, or beacon lights, artificial harbors or but few natural ones were in existence; no piers, wood or coal yards were established; and not a single village, town or city in the whole distance — where now all are conspicuous along the western shores of Lake Michigan, showing a strange contrast indeed.

It will also be remembered ... that four steamers — the *Henry Clay*, *Superior*, *Sheldon Thompson* and *William Penn* — were chartered by the United States government for the purpose of transporting troops, provisions and equipment to Chicago during the Black Hawk War, but owing to the fearful ravages made by the breaking out of the Asiatic cholera among the troops and crews on board, that two of those boats were compelled to abandon their voyage, proceeding no further than Fort Gratiot. The disease became so violent and alarming on board the *Henry Clay* that nothing like discipline could be observed — every thing in the way of subordination ceased. As soon as the steamer came to the dock, each man sprang on shore, hoping to escape from a scene so terrifying and appalling. Some fled to the fields, some to the woods, while others lay down in the streets and under the cover of the river bank, where most of them died — unwept and alone.

There were no cases of cholera causing death on board my boat until we passed the Manitou Islands [Lake Michigan]. The first person attacked died about four o'clock in the afternoon, some 30 hours before reaching Chicago. As soon as it was ascertained by the surgeon that life was extinct, the deceased was wrapped closely in his blanket, placing with some weights, secured by lashing of small cordage around the ankles, knees, waist and neck, then committed, with but little ceremony to the great deep.

This unpleasant but imperative duty was performed by the Orderly Sergeant, with a few privates, detailed for that purpose. In like manner, 12 others, including this same noble sergeant, who sickened and died in a few hours, were also thrown overboard before the balance of the troops were landed at Chicago.

The sudden and untimely death of this veteran sergeant, and his committal to a watery grave, caused a deep emotion on board among the soldiers and crew, but which I will not here attempt to describe. The effect produced upon General Scott and the other officers, in witnessing the scene, was too visible to be understood, for the dead soldier had been a very valuable man, and evidently a favorite among the officers and soldiers of the regiment.... There was one singular fact — not one of the officers of the army was attacked by the disease, while on board my ship, with such violence as to result in death, or any of the officers belonging to the boat, though nearly one fourth of the crew fell a prey to the disease on a subsequent trip, while on the passage from Detroit to Buffalo. [It appears likely the crew was exposed while stopping in Detroit.]

In the course of the day and night following [the ship's docking in Chicago], eighteen others died and were interred not far from the spot where the American Temperance House has since been erected [now corner of Lake and Wabash Avenue].... During the four days we remained at Chicago, fifty-four more died, making an aggregate of eighty-eight who paid the debt of nature. The scene of horror occasioned by this singular disease (then so little known to medical science), it would be difficult for any pen to describe, or heart to conceive, or tongue to adequately tell.[19]

Walker died in February 1865. He was particularly noteworthy for his collections of stories and events taking place during the early years of shipping on the Great Lakes. His ship, the *Sheldon Thompson*, was the first steamship on Lake Michigan.

The commander at Fort Gratiot, Major A.W. Thompson of the Second United States Infantry, was concerned enough about the presence of the sick troops that he took the measure of moving his own command from the fort to another camp on Lake St. Clair, a site about 13 miles south of Fort Gratiot. His command at the time consisted of two companies of infantry and two companies of artillery.[20] Thompson's orders had been to join General Scott, embark his troops on the steamers accompanying the general, and travel over the lakes to Fort Dearborn. But with the outbreak of disease among the troops on the steamers, Thompson was (rightly) concerned that his own men, coming in contact with the sick in the fort hospital, would also become victims of the outbreak. Thompson's decision may have helped save some lives, as there is no subsequent record of his having reported an outbreak among his men. Some of Scott's men were also quartered in the government warehouse then located on Woodbridge Street near Cass in Detroit itself. Several of these men developed the disease.

The Detroit Board of Health attempted to reassure the citizens that the outbreak was being contained:

July 10, 1832;

The committee of physicians of the Board of Health report, that so far as they have been able to ascertain, during the twenty-fours ending at 10:00

this morning, *two, and only two* (italics added), new cases of Cholera have occurred in this city; one of whom was of most inveterably intemperate and filthy habits, wandering about, from one tippling shop to another, without any fixed place of residence, or any regularity in his habits of eating and sleeping — and who had lain more than three hours after the attack, without any assistance whatever — Died in about nine hours from the attack. The habits of the other are not known to the committee.[21]

It was recommended that people remain in their homes, which in addition meant they should avoid shopping. The burden to families was significant, as food, water and other needs were often replenished daily. The importance of temperate habits was also pointed out, as it was reported that only one out of 15 people who were sober, clean or calm were at risk of the disease. Of course with a population of 3,000–4,000 people, not taking into account the surrounding region, even this low estimate meant the numbers of cases of cholera would be in the hundreds.[22] The importance of temperate habits was also emphasized by physicians dealing with the outbreak in Canada, even if the individual was unfortunate enough to develop the disease: "An intelligent and respectable physician, in allusion to the character of the cholera in Canada, gives it as his opinion that among the temperate, well-fed, well-clothed and fearless, who were attacked, the disease has been more within human control than almost any great epidemic which has ever visited our world."[23] In a way, the opinion of the physician does make sense. If the individual is well-fed and properly nourished, he might have a greater chance for survival; the disease was not 100 percent fatal.

A more unusual remedy for avoiding the cholera was reported several weeks after the epidemic had peaked: avoiding anger.

It is allowed on all hands, that anger may bring on an attack of the cholera, if the system be predisposed. A prevention of anger, therefore, is a preventive of the cholera. We have an infallible preventive, which we recommend, gratis. When you find yourself getting into a passion — no matter for what cause — immediately open this number of the Democratic Free Press, and commence the perusal of the act to establish certain post roads, etc. which begins on the first page. Read until you find yourself perfectly cool. N.B. [Note:] Persons liable to sudden attacks are recommended to keep this number of the Free Press in their pockets, or indispensables, as the case may be."[24]

Despite the attempts to allay any fears about the likelihood of infection and prevent a panic, Randall S. Rice, John Whiting, and Marshal

Chapin, members of the committee established as the Board of Health, were certainly well aware of the potential danger of an outbreak. Following the first report several weeks earlier of the presence of a different disease — smallpox — Mayor Levi Cook had issued a proclamation on June 25 to the effect that ships entering the port had first to be inspected by the Board of Health. The proclamation also applied to any ferries bringing passengers into Detroit. The Common Council of the city also allotted the sum of $1,000 to establish a hospital that could deal with any future outbreak of illness within the city.[25] The upper story as well as the jury room of the territorial courthouse located at State and Griswold streets, later to serve as the capitol building when Michigan became a state and Detroit became the first state capital, was converted into a temporary hospital in the event that an epidemic did break out in the city.

At this time in its history, the city was divided into four districts. In each of those districts citizens were designated to oversee proper sanitation procedures. The city provided bleaching powder composed of chloride of lime specifically for the purpose of disinfection in the event of an outbreak. The substance had long been used as a disinfectant and was convenient as it could either be sprinkled or used as a solution. Despite the ignorance as to the cause of cholera in 1832, when used correctly the substance could be quite effective for the desired purpose. Because of this practice, it is likely additional loss of life was averted.

The fears of the populace associated with contracting the disease were well-founded. Cholera was a devastating illness, one that could kill within hours after the first symptoms appeared. Emily Mason, the sister of Stevens Mason, Michigan's first governor, attested to the rapidity with which the illness could progress in the victim: "With this terrible cholera we lost many of our friends, and among others, our dear old 'Granny-Peg,' my mother's faithful nurse.... She died in my arms, and I went out into the night to find the 'death cart' which passed the streets day and night, calling 'Bring out the dead.'"[26] Another report related this: "One evening a charming young man from Boston sat with us on the doorstep sipping a mint julep [thought to be a preventive of the disease]. He was well, gay, at parting; by the morning he was dead."[27] In the hours prior to death the patient endured a miserable existence. A vivid description is found in a letter sent by Assistant Surgeon Samuel B. Smith to an army colleague, [Henry?] Wilson:

5. Detroit, Cholera and the Black Hawk War

The face was shrunken, as if wasted by lingering consumption; perfectly angular, and rendered particularly ghastly by the complete removal of all the soft solids, and their places supplied by dark lead lines; the hands and feet were bluish white, wrinkled as when long macerated in cold water; the eyes had fallen into the bottom of their orbs; and evinced a glaring vitality; but without mobility; and the surface of the body was cold and bedewed with an eely exudation."

The patient would lose so much fluid through dehydration that the

blood was like sludge his heart could not pump.... Such a case might begin with a diffuse but painless diarrhea that became progressively more liquid until it reached a stage where the stools resembled rice-water. Vomiting, often projectile, followed and continued even if the patient took nothing by mouth.... Bowel movements might become involuntary. As the dehydration continued, the heart began to falter and circulatory failure followed. The flow of urine decreased or stopped.... The temperature dropped below normal, the respiration became ever more rapid, and, in the final moments before death, the victim's dehydration might become so complete that even his diarrhea ceased at last."[28]

Dr. Smith died in November 1834, whether from the disease he described so vividly is unclear.

By the 18th of July the number of cases in the city had risen to 58, 28 of whom had died. By now there was no question that a significant epidemic had broken out. Nor did the weather appear to be cooperating. The heat of the Michigan summer in July, at a time in which air-conditioning was not even a dream, was particularly oppressing. And when storms appeared, heavy clouds and rain bracketed the area for several days. The city's Common Council had to appear to be doing something in response to the fear and panic among the citizenry. In the absence of an understanding of the source of the contagion, the sewage contamination of the water supply, the council ordered potash pots to be placed on many street corners in hopes that by burning pine resin and tar the process might help stop the spread of the disease. One particularly large potash kettle was placed in the intersection of Jefferson and Woodward avenues, and was kept burning both night and day. At least one young citizen later recalled that it reminded him of the fireworks held on each 4th of July.[29]

Chloride of lime, used liberally throughout the city, and smoke from the burning pine tar, blackened the skies. Many concluded that the outbreak represented some form of Divine retribution, perhaps instigated by the intemperance of the populace. Citizens of course were hoping there were measures they could take on a personal basis as means to avoid the disease. The council pointed out the usual risks associated with cholera outbreaks: avoid the drinking of "ardent spirits"; excessive eating or even poverty were risks (no remedy for poverty was suggested), as were too much sunshine, drafts, and wetness or cold at night. And "above all be fearless and you will be safe."[30] Other preventive measures included keeping the body warm, not only the feet but also the "stomach and bowels." Workmen who had no choice but to work in the cold or damp were recommended to wear wooden shoes or clogs because they were more water resistant than the leather shoes of the time. If a person had to be out at night they should return home at an early hour. The diet should primarily consist of meat or soup consisting of meat, while cold drinks should be avoided. Actually, heating a drink might also serve to kill the cholera bacillus; of course, that was not the primary purpose of the recommendation, given the lack of knowledge of the cause. If water is drunk it should be either filtered, or at least clear. Even better if the water could be mixed with brandy or absinthe. While excessive drink would have been frowned upon, and drinking brandy straight discouraged as well, apparently when diluted as a preventive the writer might overlook brandy's other properties. One is reminded of the euphemism often used in later times when alcohol might be referred to simply as "medicine" by the upper classes.

One common response to panic of course is to attempt to flee the site of the outbreak. The citizens of the city were no exception, and many did attempt to leave Detroit for the surrounding communities. The citizens there certainly did not want visitors from a place where the cholera epidemic was raging, and in response closed many of the inns or shelters where travelers might stay as they waited out events transpiring in Detroit. If travelers managed to find a place to stay they often found themselves evicted, with their luggage thrown out with them as their hosts also succumbed to the growing panic. Bridges were dismantled throughout the area to prevent travelers from passing through. Many of the towns west of Detroit such as Dearborn, Ypsilanti, Saline and others along the Sauk Trail, now Michigan Avenue/Rte. 12, had their origins as stagecoach stops. Quarantines were established outside these towns

5. Detroit, Cholera and the Black Hawk War

specifically to prevent travelers from Detroit from passing through. Among these was a guardhouse manned by Captain Josiah Burton and Lieutenant Chester Perry placed east of the town of Ypsilanti, on the route from Detroit to Chicago, some 30 miles distant. On July 10 a stage coach carrying both passengers and dispatches for General Scott at Fort Dearborn was fired upon by the guards. One horse of the four-horse team was initially thought to have been killed — it was not. The driver whipped the horse and it continued on. Once the militia, the guardians of the health of the Ypsilanti residents, realized the coach was carrying mail, they allowed it to proceed though the coach was briefly detained until it was established that the passengers carried no threat.[31] Since the coach was also carrying the mail, however, the detainment had the effect of alerting the authorities, causing a significant argument about passage of the coach. Ironically, Burton and Perry were among the petitioners several years earlier requesting that the mail route be established out of Detroit[32]; their actions of course had the effect of stopping the mail. One of the members of the militia, Lorenzo Davis, was in fact the deputy postmaster in Ypsilanti.

Since delay or stoppage of mail delivery was a legal offense, an official inquiry took place in which the incident was investigated. In August, several of the principals were requested to provide a deposition before the justice of the peace, Elias Skinner, describing their respective roles in the delay of the coach.

A local physician, S.S. Ransom, first described the quarantine requirement and his role in the incident:

> I Seth S. Ransom, of lawful age, being duly sworn, do depose and say, that under a Statute Law of the Territory aforesaid, quarantine regulations were established about the 9th of July, 1832, by the authorities of the town of Ypsilanti, in said county, prohibiting persons coming from the city of Detroit, or other supposed infected places to enter the said town of Ypsilanti until examined by a health officer; and that on the 10th day of July, 1832, affiant acted as a health officer for the purpose aforesaid, and on that day the passengers in the stage carrying the mail from Detroit west through the town of Ypsilanti were by virtue of said regulation, required to stop and be examined, previous to passing through said town — that the stage driver was distinctly informed that no one wished to detain him or the mail, but the passengers only; and affiant further saith, the stage on the 10th of July aforesaid, was requested to stop solely on account of the passengers, and no longer than was necessary for them to get out of it and be examined, which occupied

but a few minutes, not longer than is usually necessary to water the horses, and that said examination took place at a usual watering place, and further saith not.

Captain Josiah Burton, in charge of the militia at the guardhouse, then described his participation:

I, Josiah Burton ... do depose and say, that I was ordered by the authorities of the town of Ypsilanti, to carry into effect the quarantine regulations referred to in the preceding affidavit of S.S. Ransom, that in obedience to such order, I repaired to the quarantine ground about three miles east of the village of Ypsilanti [Michigan Avenue today], that on my way thither, I was particularly requested by Mark Norris, Post Master of Ypsilanti, *not to stop or delay the mail* [italics added]. That I was present every day from the 10th of July, 1832, to the 17th day of July, 1832, when the passengers were stopped from the mail coach, and it was distinctly made known to the driver that the coach driver and the mail might pass.

Not all those who were present were as compliant as the authorities might have wished. The deposition provided by Eliphalet Turner, one of the peace officers, described his role in dealing with the passengers:

I, Eliphalet Turner ... was requested by the authority of the town of Ypsilanti, to aid in enforcing the [quarantine law] and was present on the quarantine ground on the morning of the 9th of July or 10th aforesaid, together with two others without any arms or weapons, that we requested the travelers coming from Detroit to wait and be examined by the health officer. Showed them the proclamation of the Supervisor and Justices, and the quarantine law, and sent for a health officer for the purpose of examining said travelers, there being from ten to twenty, peaceably waiting for the arrival of said officer, when Samuel Stackhouse and Marcus Lane came up, said Stackhouse on being informed by said travelers of their detention, denounced the quarantine regulation, said it was all a damned piece of nonsense, that the quarantine had no right to detain travelers to go on about their business, and call at his house and get breakfast, said to one Mr. Curtis, living near, set these men (those enforcing the quarantine) to work in your cornfield — and Lane also advised said travelers to go and not be detained by the rabble [Lane's argument was that the quarantine applied only to seaports, not villages]. Said they might put all their law in force against said travelers and that he (Lane) would see them (the travelers) out of it. And this deponent further saith that the proclamation of Supervisor and Justice was exhibited in presence of said Stackhouse and Lane, and Lane said that it was Champion's [Salmon Champion, Justice of the Peace] authority, and had not law to back it up. And this deponent further saith, that he received orders from the said authorities not to detain the mail, in no case than was necessary to examine the passengers, and this deponent further saith, that he thinks if had not been for the opposition of said Stackhouse and Lane, no armed force would have been necessary to detain travelers or passengers agreeably to said quarantine regulation, as all manifested a disposition to submit to said regulation, until advised to the contrary by said Stackhouse and Lane, but after being so advised, all the said travelers except three or four, disregarded said regulation and passed along through the town of Ypsilanti. That afterward— word was sent to said authorities that more help was necessary to carry into effect said regulation, and Capt. Burton and others were sent for that purpose."[33]

Other witnesses corroborated the roles played by Stackhouse and Lane.

Perhaps not surprisingly, Marcus Lane's version of events differed from those described by the authorities on the scene. His response in the *Free Press* attempted to explain his actions:

A meeting of the inhabitants of the village of Ypsilanti (not the township) was called, in a hasty manner, on the 9th of July last. Resolutions were adopted, recommending the organization of a board of health, pursuant to a law of the last Legislative Council. I attended the meeting, and opposed the establishment of a quarantine, and consequently was subjected to the denunciation of men laboring under excited feeling. The justices and supervisors organized themselves pursuant to the resolutions agreed upon a proclamation, and handed it to Dr. A. Platt, with directions to proceed to Detroit and ascertain if the cholera was raging there, and if so, to get the proclamation printed and publish the same; but in case the cholera should be found not to prevail there, not to get the proclamation printed. Dr. Platt left for Detroit on the same evening, and arrived there on the morning of the 10th — found the cholera there — got the proclamation printed, and received the same from the office about 12:00 noon. He then started for Ypsilanti and arrived at the quarantine ground four or five hours *after* [italics added] the stage had been stopped. In your report you say "That said proclamation was, on the day of issue thereof, and immediately after, taken by some three or four of the assistants, three miles east of Ypsilanti on the Chicago Road, where it was ordered to be carried into effect. That the said proclamation was on that day there posted up and published, as well as at other places, some miles farther east on the said road." This is a new discovery, the truth of which never has been pretended. Two trials have since been had in which the question has been raised as to the publication of the proclamation, and no such evidence has been adduced; but on the contrary, Dr. Platt testified as I have before stated, and one of the men under Capt. Burton testified, that a copy of the proclamation was handed to Capt. Burton on the 10th of July (not on the day of issuing it) and taken by him to the quarantine ground, and not stuck up but carried in his pocket. You have also been deceived ...

when you say that "until Samuel Stackhouse and Marcus Lane came from the village on to the ground, and advised the persons there and others that arrived, to pay no attention to the quarantine regulations, the proclamation, or the persons issuing it, nor to those there to enforce it, but to go on." The truth is [both Stackhouse and Lane] took the stage. On our arrival at Mr. Curtiss' tavern, three miles east of Ypsilanti, we found [four gentlemen] who informed us that they were forcibly detained from going home to their families.... They asked me by what authority they were being detained, and if the persons detaining them had any such right. In answer to their inquiries I informed them that I was not aware of any proclamation being issued, and gave it as my opinion that they had no right forcibly to detain them before issuing a proclamation.[34]

Lane also had an explanation for the alleged abusive language:

I have only to say, that I was conscientious in the belief that they were pursuing an illegal and unjustifiable course; one which the law would not sanction; and that they were, many of them, trying, under the color of a discharge of duty, to gratify their malignant feelings. My life had been repeatedly threatened, and I had been an eyewitness to the shooting of the horse [actually a shot startled a horse, but none was shot], and other inhuman acts, committed by them, before a single word passed between me and the guard.[35]

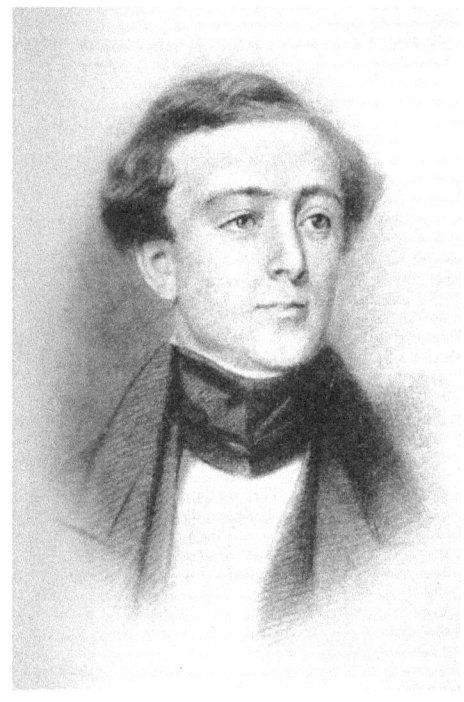

Stevens Mason, secretary of Michigan Territory and first governor (Burton, *The City of Detroit*, 1922).

Other witnesses corroborated Lane's version of events.

In summary, the chain of events associated with the mail and passenger coach appears to be as follows: On July 10 the coach left Detroit, traveling west alone the Chicago Road and reaching the east side of Ypsilanti later that morning. The coach was stopped by the authorities and the passengers were requested to disembark for an examination. Most complied, and the examination carried out by Dr. Ransom appears to have taken no more than a few minutes. Two local residents, Marcus Lane and Samuel Stackhouse, were present on the scene and took issue with the stoppage. Lane told the passengers to ignore the quarantine and proceed on their way; he appeared to have been rather abusive in his language. The premise of Lane's argument was he had not been aware that any such quarantine had been proclaimed. A shot was fired, either to stop the coach or to prevent its proceeding, though a statement to the effect that a horse had been shot was incorrect. Subsequently the stage went on its way, whether with permission or not is unclear. But the story is indicative of the situation that had developed once it became clear an outbreak of cholera was taking place in Detroit.

The end result was that the case was much ado about nothing. Deputy Postmaster Lorenzo Davis was briefly reprimanded, after which the case was dismissed.[36]

Stevens Mason, then secretary of the Michigan Territory and later first governor, ran afoul of the overzealous authorities about the same time. Mason was traveling from Detroit to Mottville in the western portion of the territory along the same road, and in order to avoid the quarantine near Ypsilanti sought the help of a friend and local surveyor, Samuel Pettibone, who might guide him along a secondary route to avoid the guards. However, a local deputy intercepted Mason and arrested him, bringing Mason before the sheriff, a Dr. Withington. After some discussion, Mason was allowed to leave.[37] Pettibone later recounted the story among his reminiscences:

> At this time I was living east of Bowen's Tavern, on the Chicago Road [now Michigan Avenue, Rt. 12 in that area] and the news of the fight with the stage [as recounted above] caused many to wish to avoid Ypsilanti, so I often acted as pilot to run them past the village. A few days after the battle, along came the [future] governor, Stevens T. Mason, on his way to Mottville. He wanted to run the guard and shun Ypsilanti. We went across the north part of the plain, crossed the Huron at the upper bridge, and came into the Chicago Road west of the village [Ypsilanti]. It was four miles to the first tavern west [present-day Saline], and only a half mile back into the village, and by going around we had not passed a tavern after leaving Sheldon's [located at the current site of Sheldon Road and Michigan Avenue]. The pressure was too great; he must go back to the village. He was arrested by

Eliphalet Turner, who brought him to the sheriff, Dr. Withington, and after a short but stormy discussion, the governor was allowed to depart, and he instantly started for Mottville. The first official act the governor was known to do was to take away the Doctor's commission as sheriff, and appoint in his stead William Anderson, of Ann Arbor.[38]

Roadblocks were set up as well in the towns north of Detroit, including the road to Pontiac. John Sheldon, the editor of the *Democratic Free Press*, Detroit's primary news source, had attempted to travel to Pontiac to engage a physician to help treat the sick in Detroit as well as the remaining soldiers at Fort Gratiot. He was stopped on the road, likely Woodward Avenue, which ran from Detroit to Pontiac by then, somewhere between Auburn and Pontiac, where he was informed by a physician who had come out to meet him that he could not even pass through the area until sufficient time had passed — at least two weeks — to demonstrate he was not a carrier of the cholera. The editor returned to Auburn, where the citizenry were sufficiently free of panic, and remained at a public house. The editor participated in a town meeting that evening during which the various options could be considered:

> Several persons expressed their sentiments in relation to the disease which had created such an alarm, and it seemed to be the general opinion of the citizens present (formed from the various facts which had been published) that the cholera was an epidemic, and was not contagious, and therefore, that it was the duty of every citizen to endeavor to calm the public alarm, and extend to the unfortunate sick all the assistance in their power. A resolution was adopted with great unanimity disapproving of the measures which had been deemed expedient by the villages of Pontiac and Rochester as calculated to produce much inconvenience to citizens who were obliged to travel, and to prevent many from obtaining medical and other assistance in case of sickness.... The alarm to which we have alluded, we should think, has in a great degree, been created and increased by the measures of security which have been adopted. The consequences of this alarmed state may well be dreaded. It will lead to a selfish and cruel abandonment of those who may be taken ill — it will induce an inhuman and inhospitable treatment of strangers — it will induce conduct which will cause lasting regret — and above all, it is one of the most active agents in multiplying cases of the dreaded disease. It is to be hoped that the considerate and calm portion of the inhabitants in every settlement, will exercise their influence and activity in arresting the unmanly and unchristian terror which exists.[39]

The village of Auburn, now the current site of Auburn Hills, was one of the few shining lights during the panic that engulfed the region.

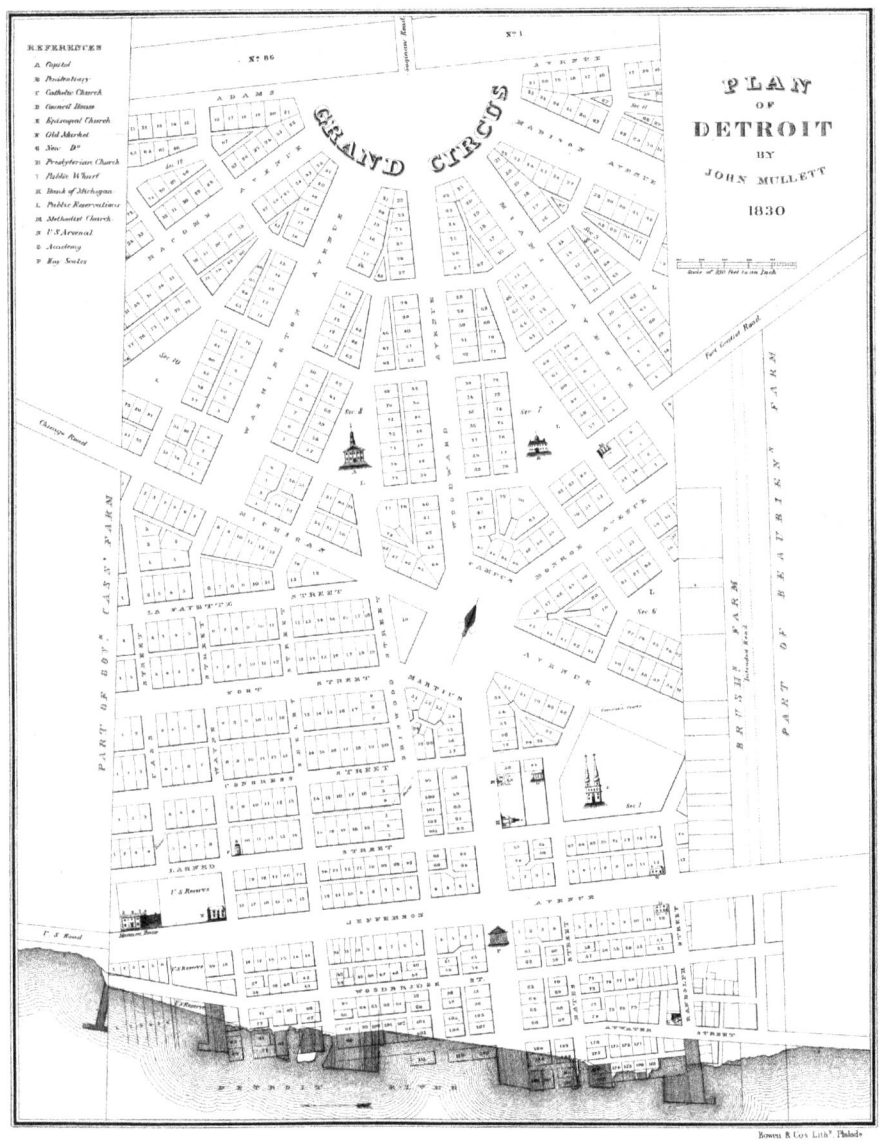

City of Detroit, 1832 (courtesy Bentley Historical Library, Ann Arbor, Michigan).

Meanwhile, for those survivors in Detroit, the epidemic was omnipresent. It was common for churches in Detroit like those elsewhere to toll their bells in response to deaths. But the numbers of persons dying in the outbreak were becoming so high that churches finally stopped their tolling, similar to what also had transpired in other cities through which cholera had passed.

A testimony to the events and panic taking place not only in Detroit but in New York as well can be found in a letter sent by Mormon founder Joseph Smith to an acquaintance, William Phelps, on July 31, 1832, reporting the observations of a visitor to Detroit during these weeks. Spelling and grammar are per the original:

> Judgment upon all the face of the earth, we have information which may be relyed upon that the cholera is cutting down its hundreds in the city of New York pr day also is raging in Boston Charleston Rochiste Albany & Buffalo and in all the large citys in the eastern country, we have Just received a letter from sister Elmira Scoba who is now at Detroit to visit her friends she states that the cholera is raging in that city to an alarming degree, hundreds of families are a fleeing to the country and the country people have become alarmed and torn up the bridges and stopped all communication and even shot peoples horses down under them who attempt to cross the river or any express two steam boats loaded with troops for the Indian expedition while going up Detroit river the cholera made its attact upon the soldiers about fifty died the rest disbanded (about six hundred in number) and the last account we have of them they could find no quarters among the inhabitants and were a dying in the sheds and fields and nobody to bury them while between us and you the Indians are a spreading death and devestation wherever they go no force has as yet been brought sufficient to stand before them frequent cases of the cholera occures on steem boats and other water crafts on the Lakes the dysentary and the Cholera Morbus are the prevailing deseases as far as our information extends and is so malignant that it baffles the skill of the most eminent Phisicians we have news from our brethren who have gone to the east God is with them pulling down the strong holds of Satan two brethren are here from the east Newhampshire & one from Vermont who are Elders and worthy young men who were brought in by the hands of Bros. Lyman Johnson & Orison Pratt who are like Peter & John building up the cause of God wherever they go and healing the sick they have baptized better then sixty since they left here we also here from many others whose good success in gaining converts to the redeemers.[40]

Potions, Myths and Treatments for Cholera

The best that can be said about most treatments available in 1832 was that at least they failed to kill the patient. Some extant treatments were described in chapter 2. It should be kept in mind, given our twenty-first century perspective, that the doctors of the time were not butchers; but neither were they aware of the causative agents for various maladies. Physician's methods were predicated on the medicine they knew, as primitive as that knowledge was. Even Louis Pasteur's understanding of the role played by microorganisms in putrefaction, a key element in development of the germ theory of disease, was still a generation in the future. Many of the methods practiced by physicians had a historical basis and were based upon what one might call superstitious behavior. If a treatment was attempted and the disease abated, the method was added to the historical literature and often reiterated. With the exception of the epidemiological work of British physician James Lind, which established the importance of fresh fruit in the prevention or cure of scurvy, nothing like a controlled study had been carried out in the study of disease by 1832.

Among the oldest treatments for disease was bleeding, the draining of small, or not so small, portions of blood. The practice had its origin in the Greek philosophers of 2,200 years previous, who linked the four humors—blood, phlegm, black bile, and yellow bile—with the four elements of earth, water, fire and air. If one was ill, or even of bad temperament, the fault was to be found in one of the humors. There were a variety of ways physicians might attempt to restore the humors, such as bleeding the patient or blood-letting through cupping, in which a vein would be cut and a hot cup placed over the wound. This would draw blood to the surface, and as the cup cooled, the vacuum would draw out the blood. This was a common method in the summer since the individual might appear red or flushed, a symptom thought to mean the presence of too much blood. Blistering might be used to remove black bile, thought to result in dryness of the mouth. Bowels might be purged or vomiting induced.

By the 1830s physicians began to focus on another symptom of diseases like cholera, inflammation. Cholera was an internal disease, but through convoluted reasoning, the symptoms of cholera—primarily the extreme diarrhea—could be attributed to internal inflammation. Cholera appeared to be most prevalent in the warmer or hot months of spring and summer, times in which because of the humidity, perspiration was inhibited. The result was an internal disruption and accumulation of blood in the internal organs. The logical treatment was to bleed the patient.

Physicians often had their own favorite treatments, some of which are described elsewhere in this book. Dr. Randall S. Rice of the Detroit Board of Health recommended a combination of bleeding and calomel (mercury chloride), a purgative. Rice declared that he actually cured patients using the calomel treatment; the reports from the subsequent 1834 outbreak in Detroit, however, indicate that all his patients ultimately died.[41] Others physicians were not as successful as Rice had declared, and as they recognized the toxicity of the substance, the technique gradually fell out of favor.[42] Some blamed diet as a cause, while recommending changes in the diet as a cure. Dr. Alvin Wood Chase, an Ann Arbor physician, wrote, "Cholera morbus arises from a diseased condition of the bile, often brought on by over-indulgence with vegetables, especially unripe fruits; usually commencing with sickness and pain at the stomach, followed by the most excruciating pain and griping of the bowels, succeeded by vomiting and purging, which soon prostrate the patient. The person finds himself unavoidably drawn into a coil by the contraction of the muscles of the abdomen and extremities." Dr. Chase's cure was to boil green beans for two hours and then eat them.[43] The number of what were obviously quack cures eventually generated their own form of humor. One "certain" cure was as follows: "Take half a pint of hen's milk, two ounces of jeesway, and mix them in a hog's horn, stirring well with a cat's feather; then roll the mass of pills as big as a piece of chalk and long as a stick, and swallow them crosswise."[44]

Whether cholera was even contagious was a point of contention among the citizenry. At least one writer from Ann Arbor at this time argued in favor of the ability of the disease to be transmitted directly from person to person. But some of the characteristics of the disease — its ability to develop in individuals with no apparent exposure, while other individuals seemingly in intimate relations with cholera victims never became ill — created understandable skepticism among those convinced other factors were involved in the spread of the disease:

> We had a hope that our citizens would not be troubled with the long arguments and facts of the cholera contagionists and non-contagionists, until the disease had wholly disappeared from the Territory. A writer in the last Ann Arbour [sic] paper has disappointed us — he has sent forward upwards of two columns, to prove that the cholera is a contagious disease, and he sup-

ports the position he has assumed by a reference to many alleged facts, all of which, however, occurred in the countries of Asia, Africa or Europe. As non-contagionists, we [i.e., the staff of the newspaper] submit for the consideration of "our adversaries" the following fact. "In a Russian village (says Captain Frankland) whose name I have forgotten, the unhappy peasantry, shut up in their miserable hovels by a sanitary cordon, seized upon two doctors who had been stationed there by the government, and whose reports they attributed their being cut off from all the sympathies and succours of humanity. The infuriated peasants tied these unlucky doctors breast to breast to the cold and livid corpses of two victims to the cholera. 'You say that the cholera is contagious; we say that it is not. If it be as you say you shall prove your words; if it be not, we have returned you good for evil, for, if you survive, you will undeceive the governor-general and make your own fortunes.' With this bitter irony, they threw the doctors into a pit dug for the bodies of the choleric dead, where they remained for two days and nights, and were at last released from their horrid prison by some charitable females who came in the night and freed them. These men did not take the cholera."[45]

Cholera's Toll

The epidemic of the disease in Detroit of course was no joke; people were dying. Prior to the 12th there were a reported 39 cases and 16 deaths, which included the seven deaths among the soldiers quartered there. The numbers from the Board of Health just for the week of July 12 provide a vivid example of the progress of the disease: July 12: nine cases, four deaths. July 13: no new cases, three deaths. July 14: three cases, one death. July 15: three cases, one death. July 16: two cases, no deaths. July 17: one case, two deaths. July 18: one case, one death.[46] The total for the period from July 4 to 19 was 58 cases and 28 deaths.

Dr. David L. Porter, a young physician in Pontiac setting up his new practice, came to Detroit during this period to investigate the outbreak. When Porter attempted to return to Pontiac, the citizens of that city refused to allow him back into his home. Porter was forced to return to Detroit until the epidemic had waned.[47] The treatment of Dr. Porter by the citizens of the village of Pontiac was in sharp contrast to the hospitality towards editor Sheldon by the village of Auburn.

Among the last victims of cholera in Detroit during the 1832 epidemic was Nathaniel Hickok. Hickok was born in 1800 in either Vermont or Connecticut, and was a sailor on a ship that had docked at Hog Island

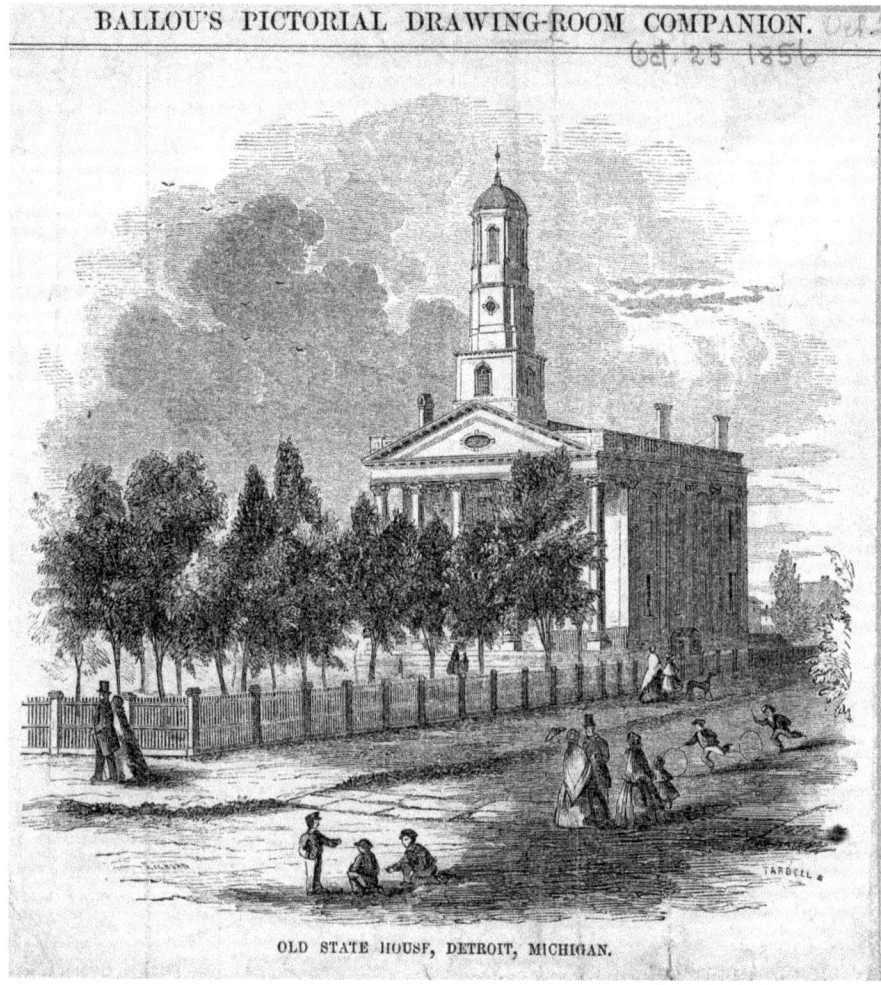

Courthouse and later capitol building, which served as a temporary hospital for cholera victims (courtesy Burton Historical Collection, Detroit Public Library).

about the end of June or beginning of July, coincident with the time during which the outbreak of cholera began in the city. Subsequently he entered the city. Whether he had already contracted cholera at the time he came to Detroit or contracted the disease after he arrived is unknown; there are some who allege he actually was the point source for the epidemic. Regardless, Hickok died of the disease on October 6 and was

5. Detroit, Cholera and the Black Hawk War

buried in the city cemetery, the current site of St. Antoine Street. Some years later in 1863 as the road was being built, most graves were removed and the bodies were reinterred in what became Elmwood Cemetery on the east side of the city, at the time located in the country. However, Hickok's grave was not disturbed and was covered in cobblestones, likely because Hickok had inscribed on his tombstone the following: "In memory of Nathaniel Hickok, who died of Cholera October 6, 1832. Good friend, for Jesu's sake forbear to dig the dust enclosed here. Blest be he that spares these stones, and curst be he that moves my bones." Most of the laborers being highly superstitious, they refused to move the body and arguments lasted for weeks, as nobody could be induced to disturb the gravesite. Finally an itinerate laborer was paid with whiskey and some extra cash to remove Hickok's grave and rebury the bones in Elmwood Cemetery.

The early nineteenth century was a period of religious revival. Church membership was in the ascendancy, and particularly on the fringes of civilization such as in Detroit, religious zealotry was making its periodic appearance. One common belief was the theocratic origin of disease, the idea that epidemics such as the one taking place were the result of an angry God meting out some form of punishment. And if God had been behind the outbreak, it was logical to assume he could end it as well. On July 12 the *Democratic Free Press* reported that the Presbytery of Detroit had recommended "to the churches under their care, the observance of Thursday, the 19th inst. as a day of humiliation and special prayer to God, that He would avert the pestilence from our

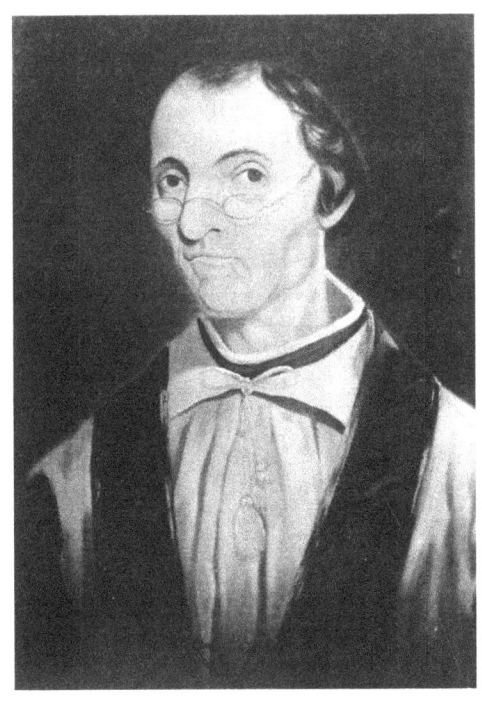

Gabriel Richard (courtesy Burton Historical Collection, Detroit Public Library).

land, and, in the midst of deserved wrath, remember mercy."[48] The date was accepted and a day of humiliation and prayer took place on the 19th. That same day the Common Council lifted the quarantine, allowing business to return to a semblance of normal.

Perhaps the most prominent member of the city to succumb to cholera in the current epidemic was Father Gabriel Richard (1767–1832), the Catholic priest and among the most important clergy in the territory. Father Gabriel first came to Detroit in 1798 as assistant pastor at St. Anne's Church. In addition to a school he established there, he was among the founders of what became the University of Michigan, and was serving on the board of trustees for that institution at the time of his death. His death was a direct result of ministering to the victims of the disease during the outbreak:

> He had no fear of the disease while attending those just ready to be borne to their long homes, and such was his anxiety for his parishioners that he utterly neglected his own health and he finally sunk under his exertions and the debilitating effects of diarrhea. The disease assumed an alarming appearance on the 9th, and the deceased, though suffering little pain, continued to grow worse, until the 12th, when he was told by the Reverend Mr. Badin, that his end was near. He expressed his willingness to die, and wished that the blessed Sacrament might be administered, and immediately after he uttered these words — *nunc dimittis servum tuum Domine, secundum verbum tuum in pace* [Now Lord, you can let your servant go in peace]. Shortly after he was asked if the extreme unction should be administered; he gave a silent consent, and seemed to long to be with his blessed Savior. His pulse continued to beat until 10 minutes past three o'clock A.M. when his soul, tired and disgusting with the affairs of this fleeting world, winged its way to Him who gave it, and left the church to mourn the loss of one of her most learned Bishops.[49]

He was laid to rest in St. Anne's Church.

It has been suggested it was not the cholera to which the priest had succumbed, but rather exhaustion. Certainly at the age of 65 and after a hard and challenging life, exhaustion would be understandable. He had appeared to be in good health, even presiding at a wedding ceremony a month earlier. However, the symptoms described in the obituary that appeared in the *Democratic Free Press* were consistent with those of cholera; the strong likelihood is that he died from that disease, combined with the encumbrances of old age.[50]

Others of prominence who died from cholera in Detroit during this

5. Detroit, Cholera and the Black Hawk War

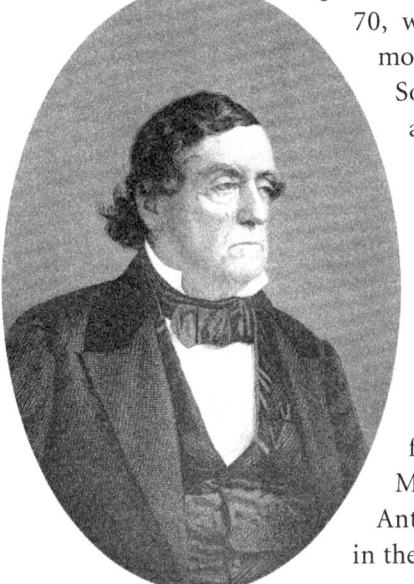

Lewis Cass, secretary of war (1831–1836) (Burton, 1922).

period included Mrs. Katherine Sproat, age 70, who died on July 15. She was the mother of Mrs. Judge Solomon Sibley. Solomon Sibley was an important attorney and politician in the Michigan Territory, becoming chief justice of the territorial, and then state, supreme court. Elizabeth Cass, the daughter of Governor Lewis Cass, died that same day, though whether from cholera or another affliction was not clear. Mrs. Mary Trowbridge, wife of James Trowbridge from Cincinnati, died on August 8. Mrs. Catherine Dequindre, wife of Antoine Dequindre, a prominent figure in the city and veteran of the War of 1812, died on September 13. These victims, along with Father Gabriel, were among the last to die as a result of the current epidemic. By the end of July the city no longer reported the number of victims in the outbreak.

Elsewhere the disease began to disappear as well. The total dead from the seven-week epidemic in Detroit appears to have been fewer than 60, though estimates have proposed numbers approaching 100; likely these have included persons dying from other causes during this period. Detroit was fortunate in being spared the worst of the epidemic — this time. In contrast, over 3,500 persons died in New York City. The disease had ranged as far as areas west of Lake Michigan, in what is now the state of Wisconsin. But while most cities of substantial size had encountered the disease, there were still a few that avoided the epidemic, including Charleston and Boston. They likely avoided the worst of the epidemic because they implemented both quarantine and sanitary procedures.

6

Cholera Returns: 1834

The death of Father Gabriel Richard during September 1832 was part of the final chapter of the outbreak that year. For the next two years cholera appeared to disappear from the Michigan Territory, and the disease was largely forgotten in the day-to-day lives of the people. The population of the city doubled over those next two years to nearly 5,000 persons as travelers continued to settle in the region, attracted by the expanses of open land throughout the territory. Nearly 500 homes and dwellings could be found within the city limits, taxing an already overburdened sanitation system; the "Grand Sewer," which would alleviate some of the problem associated with the waste, would not be built for another two years. In the middle of July 1834 cholera again appeared, and during the next eight weeks it struck the city with what can only be described as a vengeance, as if it were attempting to make up for the relatively moderate epidemic of the two years previous. The source of this outbreak, unlike that of the previous two years, would not be precisely pinpointed. That 1832 epidemic spread not only into Illinois, but down the Mississippi River as far as New Orleans, where it remained endemic to the city. Likewise, the population in New York State continued to report cases of the disease. One can easily conjecture that travelers from any of these regions could have brought the disease back to Detroit. Coincident with the outbreak that August in Detroit was a similar outbreak of cholera in Sandusky, Ohio. The source of the Sandusky epidemic may have been a traveler from Detroit named Childs, who reportedly became ill and died from the disease soon after arriving in Sandusky with the intent of working at a local shipyard. The outbreak subsequently spread through the citizenry of that town.[1]

Among the first victims of this new 1834 outbreak was the surprise illness and death of the territorial governor, General George Porter (1791–1834) on July 6. The obituary highlighted his career, but whether to avoid

6. Cholera Returns: 1834

concern among the citizenry or because of ignorance of the events surrounding his death, it never referred to cholera as the cause: "We send forth our sheet today, clad in the sad weeds of woe, in respect to the memory of General George B. Porter, late Governor of the Territory of Michigan. He died on Sabbath last after an illness of only four days. General Porter at the time of his death was in the forty third year of his age and on Tuesday last in the full enjoyment of his health attending, as was his wont, with assiduously to the discharge of his official duties."[2]

Porter had come from a family steeped in both politics and the military. His father, Andrew Porter, had been a general during the Revolutionary War. Porter himself had been a major during the War of 1812. A brother, David, later served as governor of Pennsylvania, and another brother, James Madison Porter, served as secretary of war under President John Tyler during the 1840s. George Porter had been territorial governor during the cholera outbreak in 1832, but escaped the illness at that time. Prior to his illness and death, Porter had been building a brick home in the Springwells section of Detroit. Replacing Porter as governor was Stevens Mason, who became known as the "boy governor" as he was only 20 years old at the time he replaced Porter.

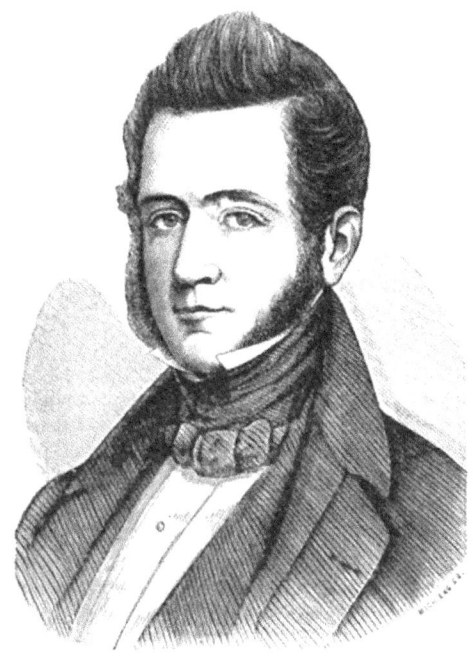

General George Porter, territorial governor of Michigan, who succumbed to cholera during the 1834 epidemic (courtesy Bentley Historical Library, Ann Arbor, Michigan).

The mayor of Detroit during the beginning of the 1834 outbreak was Charles Trowbridge. The challenge before the mayor was not only how best to deal with the epidemic, but how to prevent the panic that was sure to follow; the citizens who had been living in Detroit two years earlier were aware of the potential devastation inherent in the disease and had no desire to deal with it a second time. As the epidemic developed it quickly became clear that it was no respecter of social class; the myth commonly associated with cholera was that it was primarily a disease of intemperance, or at least associated with the lower social classes. Not this time: "The alarm that spread all over Detroit was created and extended not merely by the sudden and awful deaths which occurred on the steamers, on the docks, among the woodpiles and the merchandise strewed along the river, not merely among the laboring, the dissipated, the filthy and reckless portion of the community, but by the deaths among the most temperate, the most cleanly and apparently among the most calm and courageous."[3]

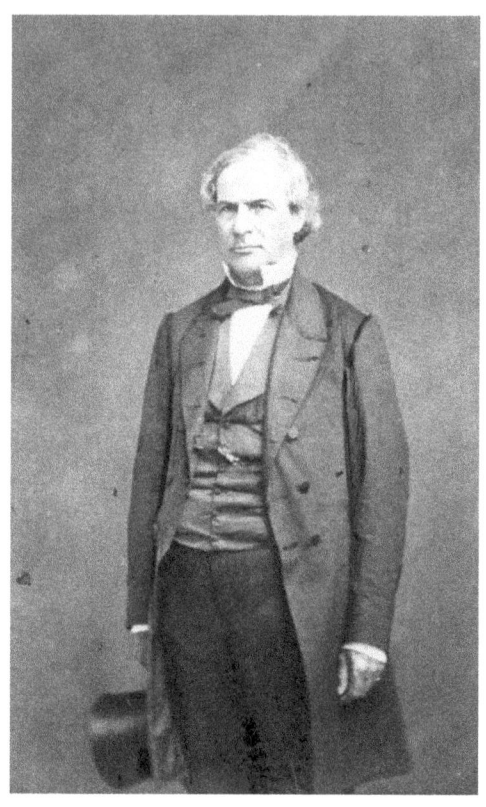

Charles Trowbridge, mayor of Detroit, 1834 (courtesy Burton Historical Collection, Detroit Public Library).

By the second week of August 1834 there were 49 deaths reported from the disease, some of which were attributed to the "imprudent use of cold water, when the blood was much heated." Twenty-eight additional deaths were attributed to other diseases.[4] The newspaper complained that the authorities were providing little information to the public regarding the outbreak:

> The public have, as yet, possessed no means of obtaining any definite information respecting the prevalence of Cholera among us—consequently an undue excitement has been created, giving rise to false or highly exaggerated reports.

6. Cholera Returns: 1834

Physicians of intelligence assure us, confidently, that although there have been cases of Cholera, the disease cannot be considered as an epidemic. No instance has yet occurred without a premonitory diarrhea of several hours duration. Imprudence in diet, drinking cold water [perhaps the actual source of the infection] in a heated condition of blood, and the excessive use of ardent spirits have been the principal predisposing causes. The physicians advise an entire abstinence from corn, cucumbers, new potatoes and all other vegetables in any degree crude; also from medicine except when directed and administered by a physician. The best advice which we can give is, to keep cool.[5]

The assurance to the citizenry that no epidemic was in progress belied the events taking place in front of them; if nearly 60 deaths from cholera in two weeks was not an epidemic one wonders how else they would define such an outbreak. Some of the vitriol was reserved for the Common Council, which, like administrative bodies anywhere and at any time, was accused of not doing enough to contain the outbreak:

The want of energy and action on the part of our city authorities and the seeming apathy manifested by them to the cleanliness of our streets, demand from us some notice. The contrast between the present board of Aldermen, and the Board of 1832, when cholera was raging among us with such malignity, is so plain, that it cannot escape observation. Then, a rigorous and efficient police was established. A Board of Health was formed, and daily and correct reports were made, and the public were truly informed of every thing in relation to the existence of sickness among us. Now, all is left to surmise — the few panic-stricken and weak minded are allowed to tell their own surmises, as matters of fact, creating a most appalling sensation abroad. Then, street commissioners were selected in every part of the city. The streets were kept clean and dry, and not so now, after a shower was the water standing in large pools in every part of the city. There appears to be a total neglect of this important part of the duties of the now Common Council, driving the present prevalence of the cholera among us. Nuisances of every description, we are told are to be found in every part of the city, and yet no efficient means are adopted for their suppression.[6]

The Common Council through a different source, the *Detroit Journal*, was fast to respond, calling these accusations "manifestly unfounded and unjust." The editor of the *Democratic Free Press* chose at the same time to reply to the *Journal's* rebuttal for each of the five issues:

The editor of the *Journal* examined the records of the Common Council and found: 1st. That more attention has been paid to the removal of nuisances, by that body, since their election in April, than had been paid for years before.

...Will the honorable member of the Common Council, who furnished Major [Thomas] Rowland with this fact, point out the places where this attention has been bestowed. It certainly cannot be found in the improvement of the streets, or in the abatement of nuisances in any part of the city, under his inspection or any other member of the board: and it is of this, that we, in common with a large majority of our fellow-citizens, complain.

2nd. That more money has been expended within four months, for this object, than for the two years previous, or than in 1832.

If this Common Council had expended more money within four months, than for two years previous, or than in 1832, (during the prevalence of the same malady) they are that much more liable to censure ... as it is evident that little or nothing has been done, where it was most needed, towards improving the health of the place. And will the same member of the Common Council inform the public through his mouth-piece, where all this money has been expended ... It is admitted, by a large majority of citizens, that the whole city was never known to be in a more filthy condition—and by strangers, that "in all their travels, they have found no place of its size, where so little attention is paid to public cleanliness."

With regard to the third article of defense, in the *Journal*, it is, perhaps, wrong to impute blame to the Common Council, for the negligence of the Physicians, and their inability to compel them to make reports.

As to the fourth article, we make the same reply as to a previous assertion, that the committees in each of the four districts, ought to have left some evidence of their doings: And why was it not in the power of the Common Council, as well as for private citizens, to procure laborers: for we have seen men, not a few, engaged in ditching and draining in various parts of the city, on private account.

"5th. We are informed that it is not a fact that the Council ordered the chloride of lime to be locked up and sold as stated in one of our city papers, and that none has been sold except in one instance for private purposes.

"It may be a fact that the Council did not order the lime to be sold; but it is a fact, as we are assured by one of our most respectable citizens, that he was told by the marshal that 'the lime could not be had to abate private nuisances, unless an account of it was kept.'

"We believe with the *Journal*, that it is incumbent upon every householder to look carefully to his own premises, and we have no doubt that such is the case. There is no cause of complaint on that score, but it is of the disgraceful appearance of our most public streets and lanes. Jefferson Avenue, a street capable of being made as clean as a floor has been in a shocking condition the last two or three months: and all that the Common Council can boast of having done, as far as we can discover, is, to have scattered a few bushels of lime about several of the principal streets—the result of unceasing importunity on the part of the citizens.[7]

6. Cholera Returns: 1834

There was of course no shortage of new ideas as to how best to treat victims of the disease. Even Randall Rice, the physician and member of the Board of Health in 1832, was forced to acknowledge that his treatment, which consisted of bleeding and calomel, provided no benefit, though whether he conceded his method actually contributed to the death is unlikely. One treatment that might actually have provided some relief was described in a letter sent from Mexico to a local Detroit doctor:

> In New Orleans, they learnt to treat the Cholera so successfully, as to drive off its terrors, and it is well to know the mode in case it should return to Detroit. The recipe is as follows: take, of rectified camphor, pulverized, one fourth of a drachm, one scruple of calomel, one drachm of cayenne pepper, and pulverized gum Arabic sufficient to make into a mass, and make the whole into twelve pills. Take five of these pills, and put yourself under a couple of blankets, and drink warm chamomile tea, a little at a time. If the heat is not restored generally to the system, the feet, ankles, hands and wrist and spine must be rubbed hard, under the blankets, and with red pepper and whiskey, or some stimulating ointment, by four persons, in order that it be done speedily, and continued without intermission, until a warm sweat is produced over the whole body. When this is done, cover up, and drink the chamomile tea in small quantities, as the patient may require; and after he has perspired sufficiently, which will be known by the heat subsiding gradually, change his flannel and linen, and rub him dry with flannel, moistened in whiskey; put him between dry sheets and let him go to sleep. In robust habits, give two pills three or four hours after the dose. As soon as the premonitory symptom (diarrhea) appears, give five of the pills immediately. To check this, some give five grains of calomel, and one of opium, instead of the above pills, and repeat the dose in four or five hours, if necessary. I have been this particular, because of the efficacy of this remedy, and of the apprehension that the cholera will linger for some years in the United States.[8]

Other than the calomel, a mercury derivative, the remainder of the recipe would likely do no harm, and replacing lost fluids with chamomile tea might have benefited the patient. During the cholera epidemic of 1832 some 4,300 persons died in New Orleans. The writer's contention that "in New Orleans, they learnt to treat the Cholera so successfully, as to drive off its terrors" might be subject to disagreement.

A more popular cure appeared at the same time: liberal use of alcohol. The lower social classes drank whatever was available. If you were part of the monied class, port wine was the drink of choice. Women might spike their daily flagroot tea, an ancient aromatic sometimes used as a treatment for disease, with a little brandy. Male members of the higher social class often gathered in the reception and drinking rooms — not the same sites in the building, but they very well could have been mistaken for such — of the Mansion House hotel. Since brandy had been prescribed by two of the leading physicians in the city, Drs. Rice and Whiting, men could stand around and discuss the issues of the day while imbibing what they could convince themselves was "medicine" that could ward off the disease. In fact Dr. Silas Spencer of Detroit concocted a variation of the brandy "cure": "He fed his patients freely with warm brandy sling infused with pepper-sauce, laudanum [opium — Was there a cholera cure which did not contain either a narcotic or alcohol?], essence of peppermint and spirits of hartshorn, keeping them at the same time at oven heat with hot bricks."[9] If they wished for reality to impose itself in their thoughts or discussions of social issues they had only to stand in the gallery and look down the street, where they could observe carts or carriages carrying the newly dead, many on their way to the cemetery. The Mansion House, including the bar, was run by one Mrs. Joshua Boyer. Upon her death, likely from cholera during the epidemic, the building was emptied of its occupants. Early the following year the old hotel was sold by her husband.

Meanwhile the epidemic showed no evidence of having peaked. By August 20 there were a reported 222 victims.

The Common Council might have been lax in developing a means to control the epidemic, but the city's physicians were not. Some, such as Drs. Randall Rice and Marshall Chapin, had been through this before, two years earlier. Others who began to organize a fledgling medical society during these years included Drs. Douglass Houghton and Zina Pitcher, at one time a partner in practice with Rice, Ebenezer Hurd, Robert McMillan, Arthur Porter, J.B. Scovill, N.B. Stebbins and Lewis Starkey.[10] Starkey had another connection with Detroit's long history in an additional area: baseball. Lewis Starkey's son, Henry Starkey, was one of the founding members of the Franklins, the first baseball club organized in the city of Detroit and the first club in the West to play by what were known as the (New York) Knickerbocker Rules, the forerunner of today's baseball rules. Most of the members of the team were employed at the *Free Press*; the team initially played on a field located at the corner of Beaubien and High streets, later moving to a site on Woodward

6. Cholera Returns: 1834

Avenue. The Starkey family moved to Detroit from Binghamton, New York, in 1833, settling for a time in Detroit, where Lewis established a medical practice. They subsequently moved to Kalamazoo, from where Lewis later served in the state senate. Henry was trained as a printer, a job he left upon enlisting for the Mexican War in 1846. After the war Henry returned to Detroit, eventually becoming city editor for the *Free Press*.[11]

Dr. Zina Pitcher (1797–1872), in addition to being a physician, was also a major political figure in the city, twice serving as mayor (1840, 1841 and 1843). Pitcher was a founding member of the Wayne County Medical Society, serving for a time as its president. Between 1837 and 1852 he was a regent of the University of Michigan and was instrumental in developing the medical school there. Pitcher was a strong proponent as well of quality education for young people, and on his initiative the city of Detroit established free public schools.

Dr. Ebenezer Hurd was also an ardent abolitionist. A story later related by his daughter described one episode in which he demonstrated his bravery:

> One summer evening in 1858 Dr. Hurd's daughter Elizabeth was crossing the railroad bridge which spans the avenue at Dequindre Street. Suddenly a colored man of herculean build emerged on the bridge from the abutment below and, pointing across the [Detroit] river said, "I want to get over there. I want to be free." Elizabeth went home and informed her father, who immediately put on his hat and coat and sallied forth. He took the fugitive up the river to Pitts Lumber Yard and procured a boat. The fugitive said he could row. He pulled out of the slip with superhuman energy and the boat went swiftly across the river. The doctor watched the boat until it was out of sight, and went home with the consciousness of a good deed well done.[12]

Dr. Hurd's brother, Gildersleeve Hurd, once owned the land on which the University of Detroit now stands. Hurd never attended medical school, but learned his profession as an apprentice to others. It appears he had as much success in dealing with the disease as anyone could with the limited understanding and resources of the time. Unfortunately one person he was unable to save was a favorite servant girl from River Rouge; she was only 20.

Dr. Houghton (1809–1845) was an experienced physician, but he had also been trained in geology; Houghton had been among the first to explore the Keweenaw Peninsula in upper Michigan. In 1837 he was appointed by Governor Stevens Mason as the state geologist. He was also the first professor of geology at the University of Michigan. After brief service as mayor of Detroit (1842), he continued his interests as a surveyor in the unexplored regions of the northern peninsula. In 1845 he was drowned while working on a survey near Lake Superior.

Prominent Detroit Victims During the 1834 Outbreak

The worst single day during the epidemic was August 26, when 36 persons were reported to have died. General Charles Larned was among those who fell victim to the disease that week. Larned had been a member of the regiment massacred by the British and their Native American allies in what was known as the River Raisin massacre near Monroe, Michigan, during the War of 1812. Surviving, Larned gained a measure of revenge in the Battle of the Thames later in the war, during which the native leader Tecumseh was killed. Following the war Larned established a law practice in Detroit, later serving as attorney general of the Michigan Territory under Governor George Porter. His residence and office were located at Woodward Avenue and what is now Larned Street, the site being named for Charles Larned.

Larned had been present during the cholera outbreak in 1832, again emerging without having become infected. In 1834 his fortune ran out. During the outbreak he worked tirelessly trying to help others, even spending days and nights without sleep. Unfortunately he was exposed to the agent, either while ministering to the ill or through drinking contaminated water, and died from the disease on August 13. Members of the 1st Brigade, of which he had been a respected commanding general, wore mourning crepe on their left arms for 30 days. Among those whom Larned had been attending at the times of their deaths was Governor Porter, who had succumbed the previous month. Larned had also been a member of the committee established to make the arrangements for Porter's funeral. His friends recalled not only his efforts in helping the less fortunate, but his singular mode of dress. Considered a strikingly handsome man, Larned was usually attired in a dark blue coat with brass buttons, silk pants and hat, and a watch fob with seals that signaled his approach before he was even seen.[13]

6. Cholera Returns: 1834

Thomas Knapp, a well-known member of the community and former Wayne County sheriff, was a victim. Knapp was an unwilling participant in what had been the last execution under Michigan law. Stephen Simmons, a local tavern keeper, was convicted in 1830 of the murder of his wife, and was sentenced to be hanged. Knapp, as the sheriff, had the task of directing the execution. Knapp had been a devout member of Detroit's Methodist Episcopal Church, and became increasingly uncomfortable with having Simmons' blood on his hands. There were likely other influences as well. Knapp was a political appointee not likely to survive in that position more than a few additional months. Since his tenure as sheriff was limited and preferring not to have to deal with the execution, Knapp resigned two weeks before the scheduled execution date.[14] Knapp left a widow and two children, and a home noteworthy for its beautiful shrubs and flowers.

Other deaths that week from cholera included Francis P. Browning, who owned a hardware store on Jefferson Avenue and had been elected as commissioner of district schools. Browning was considered one of the most prominent citizens in Detroit at the time of his death. Among his contributions was his instrumental role in the donation of the lot for the Baptist Church, of which he was a member, in 1828. Browning had built one of the more impressive homes of the period at the corner of Griswold and Larned streets. He was also known as a prominent abolitionist.

Ebenezer (Eb) Canning, a lover of English literature and the arts, had been a graduate of Williams College in Massachusetts several years earlier. He had won a number of competitions in literature while in college, and following his graduation had published works in a number of the prominent magazines of the time. After teaching classical works at a private school, Canning obtained a position as midshipman's tutor on the frigate *United States*, gaining an opportunity to travel to the Mediterranean:

> After visiting every port of importance in the Mediterranean, gazing upon the ruins of ancient cities, feasting his soul in the paradise of Italy, and storing his mind with the rich imagery of Greece, Spain, Africa, and the Levant, thus connecting the presence with his rich recollections of the past, he returned home in August 1833.
>
> After visiting his parents and remaining a few weeks in his native village,

on the banks of the Connecticut, he took his leave and came to this Territory—never to return! For about nine months past he has acted as associate editor of the *Detroit Courier*, though his name did not appear as such. The poetic effusions which have appeared in that paper over the signature "Z" as also much of the editorial matter, was from his pen. His death was extremely sudden and unexpected.[15]

Mary Witherell was the wife of Benjamin Witherell, a prominent jurist in Detroit. She left four surviving children in addition to her husband.

Just removal of the dead became a challenge, as citizens of the city fled in panic much as they had two years previously: "To obtain nurses at night and aids and assistants to remove and bury the dead became almost impossible. Despair was fast settling upon all who remained. The stages were loaded down each succeeding morning with load after load of frightened people, who fled in terror to Pontiac, to Ann Arbor, to Jackson or Monroe, and who not unfrequently died on their way, or immediately after reaching their destination of supposed safety."[16]

Most of the deaths, of course, rather than being among the prominent members of the city as described above, were of the largely anonymous victims characteristic of epidemics throughout history. Many left behind families: "By the blessing of divine Providence, we are all well except Mother, but she is much better than when William left.... The cholera is spreading about the county above and below town [Detroit].... No less than fourteen had died out of the late Parlitey [sic] family including the family on his farm below town. It is believed that this disease has proved more fatal this year than last, and finally almost everything would turn into cholera."[17]

The Work of Father Martin Kundig

One noteworthy figure during the epidemic was Father Martin Kundig (1805–1879). Kundig was born in Switzerland, and after serving in Rome with the Swiss Papal Guard, came to Michigan in 1833 as a member of the Catholic Diocese of Detroit. The diocese had a large number of German-speaking Catholics, many of whom were unable to understand the current services conducted by a French priest. Father Kundig was fluent in four languages: French, German, Italian and

6. Cholera Returns: 1834

English, and appeared an ideal choice for tending to the immigrant flock. Kundig had already established himself in the community when the epidemic of 1834 took place. In March 1832 the county supervisors had established a committee to decide upon a location for the first county poorhouse. The commission was provided $1200, and later that month land was purchased in the township of Hamtramck, now the corner of Gratiot Avenue and Mount Elliott, but in 1832 some two miles outside the city of Detroit. A two-story frame house was built on the site. The first administrator of the site, J.P. Cooley, lasted a little over a year, and in 1834 Father Kundig replaced Cooley as superintendent; he was placed in charge of all administration of the program.

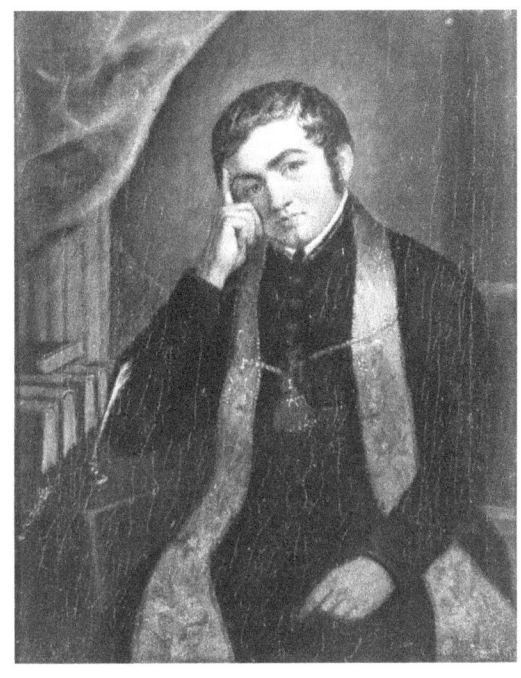

Father Martin Kundig (courtesy Burton Historical Collection, Detroit Public Library).

Kundig already had a level of medical training, and while not a physician, had a basic knowledge in the treatment of cholera. A cholera hospital was set up in the First Presbyterian Church on August 9 by local Catholics who had recently purchased the building. Every other pew was removed to allow for beds to be placed in the aisles, and a partition through the middle allowed for the separation of the sexes. Much of the work was through the local Catholic Female Association (Sisters of St. Clare).

It was reported that Father Kundig visited every bedside in every house in which cholera appeared, paying particular care to the children, many of whom were now orphans. He personally carried many of the sick to the hospital, where they might receive at least a minimum of care. Elsewhere, some of the cholera victims were removed from passing ships and simply left on the wharves, or would be found lying in the alleys. When Father Kundig found these unfortunate persons he carefully placed them in the wagon he used for transportation, and brought them to the former church, which now served as a hospital. Kundig was not the only individual collecting and bringing victims to the hospital. At least one other person, an Irish laborer named John Canann, was also employed for this purpose. Part of Canann's job was even more grisly, to remove any bodies of those who had died from the cholera. On at least one occasion Canann was rather overzealous in carrying out his work. While loading the dead on his cart for the trip to the cemetery, Canann realized one of the "bodies," a man named Rider, was still alive. That didn't deter Canann from his job, and he continued to attempt to load the man on his cart despite protestations on the part of the clearly ill victim. Canann's response was that it made no difference anyway, as Rider would be dead before they reached the cemetery. Nevertheless, Rider did survive, and was still living as late as 1860.[18]

To say the city was stingy with its monetary resources is to put it mildly. Father Kundig was given 16 cents a day per patient to pay for food and clothing, a sum that eventually was raised to 22 cents. The sum total of the allocation provided by the city to Father Kundig during the epidemic came to slightly more than $1,350, which was not only for food and clothing, but also for additional merchandise and even coffins and payment to the grave diggers.

The original poorhouse proved far from adequate in the care of orphaned children, and Father Kundig purchased the adjacent site of land, erecting a second home for the orphans; the purchase was made with his own money. Many of the approximately 100 children were destitute, and some 60 were bedridden. Kundig was forced at one point to feed them with potatoes purchased at $1.25 per bushel.

An appropriation of $3,000 requested by Governor Mason helped relieve some of Kundig's financial burdens. Nevertheless, he still owed creditors thousands of dollars and was forced to repay them out of his own funds. Kundig sold his books and even the guitar he had brought with him from Switzerland. After many years, however, Kundig was able to repay his creditors.[19] Kundig served as superintendent of the poorhouse until April 1839; at that time it was moved to Nankin township into a log house once known as the Black Horse Tavern.[20]

6. Cholera Returns: 1834

Father Kundig continued to have an impact on victims of cholera, with particular emphasis on those children who were orphaned. He moved to Milwaukee during the 1840s, and was there during the 1849 outbreak. As the story was related, a woman with seven sons and who was dying of cholera requested Father Kundig to take them in his charge. He did so, and with the aid of his two sisters brought them to live in his home. Milwaukee's bishop, John Henni, became aware of the children's plight, and established St. Aemilian as a home for orphan boys. The orphanage continues to exist today. Even long after his death, Kundig continued to be referred to as "The Apostle of Charity in Detroit."[21]

The epidemic appeared to have abated by the end of August. The grisly death count for the week ending on September 10 was four, and even those had taken place earlier that week; no deaths were reported for the previous few days. At that time the newspapers stopped reporting a weekly death toll, declaring the epidemic to be over. The estimate for total fatalities was somewhat over 320 deaths for the previous eight or so weeks, though numbers vary. The precise level of mortality is unknown, but estimates are that the epidemic killed between 7 and 10 percent of the population. Given the census number of approximately 4,900, this would translate to between 340 and 500 deaths. Within the level of error, the estimate of 320 deaths may be a reasonably accurate figure. Seventy-five of those deaths were of children.

With the declaration of an end to the epidemic, life began a return to normal. One of the first facets of that normality was the reopening of the theater, which took place in Colonel David McKinstry's entertainment center, also known as the Michigan Garden. The entertainment center was located on Randolph Street near Fort. One of the first performances, held on September 18, was *Black-eyed Susan*, starring a Mrs. Barstow: "Mrs. Barstow respectfully informs the Ladies and Gentlemen of Detroit and its vicinity that the managers have generously offered her, and set apart tomorrow evening, September 18 for her benefit; on which occasion will be presented the melodrama, entitled the *Blind Man*, and the nautical Drama called *Black-eyed Susan* (by desire) with other entertainers, for which refer to bills of the day."[22] The local theater critic had much to say about the opening of the play, as well as comments about the deportment of the younger crowd: "I would humbly suggest to some portions of the audience, that though they pay for the pleasure of edifying their fellow auditors with sundry horselaughs, still they should have respect enough for the author, the actors and the audience, not to interrupt the best scenes in the tragedy. We would also suggest to the gentlemen whose bounden duty is to keep order, that there are nightly some twenty boys in the gallery including 'dead-heads' who evince a more laudable desire to 'split the ears of the groundlings.'"[23]

The performance on the 18th appears to have been a success, and the theater-goers were in a happy mood as they left the theater. However, reality quickly intruded. While heading towards their homes they encountered the sexton, Israel Noble, riding on his horse while leading a half-dozen carts and drays loaded with dead bodies. Noble, who was also a steward in the Mechanics' Society, one of Detroit's charitable institutions, suggested they close the theater and wait another day, out of respect for the dead.[24]

David McKinstry (1778–1856), also known as Detroit's "Amusement King," was one of Detroit's more colorful figures, now largely forgotten, from that bygone era. McKinstry came to Detroit in 1815 with nothing but a wife, four children and a lot of ambition. After becoming a member of the fire department, his work ethic resulted in his being appointed to the post of inspector of the Port of Detroit. His work came to the attention of Lewis Cass, the territorial governor, who appointed him as a commissioner on several road projects, including that of the Saginaw Road from Pontiac to Saginaw (now portions of U.S. 24 and Dixie Highway). As a contractor, McKinstry was instrumental in the construction of the state capitol building. But it was in the field of entertainment that many of his most notable contributions would be found. After purchasing the Methodist Church, located at the intersection of Gratiot and Library avenues, he converted the building into a theater, the first in Detroit. It was this theater in which the play described above was performed that September at the close of the epidemic.

McKinstry's entertainment holdings in downtown Detroit included a museum of "oddities," located at Jefferson Avenue and Griswold, and the circus and menagerie at Library and Gratiot. Several years later McKinstry placed his collection of wooden bathtubs in a building across from his amusement center; one could bathe while listening to a band concert.[25] McKinstry spent the last years of his life living in Ypsilanti.

6. Cholera Returns: 1834

Despite the criticism leveled at the Common Council, the city appears to have been better prepared in dealing with the outbreak than it had been two years previously. Several sites were established as hospitals, and a small army of volunteers and physicians did what they could, despite resources being limited. On October 20, Stevens Mason, secretary and acting governor of the territory, proclaimed Thursday, November 27, "a day of public thanksgiving and prayer; that contemplating with reverence and resignations, the dispensations of the Supreme Ruler of the Universe, in the destructive pestilence which has visited our Territory, we may present our prayers of gratitude, for being permitted still to enjoy a participation in the blessings of his providence."[26]

That the territorial governor would invoke a role played by "Divine Providence" in both the outbreak of cholera and its subsequent disappearance was not unusual for the times. The 1830s represented what has been called the Second Great Awakening, a religious revival in which missionaries and others of similar zeal spearheaded a national movement to "Christianize" the population. Some of the messages were to play significant roles in coming decades; the development of the abolitionist movement was to a large degree the product of the same religious revivalism. However, in order to justify the presence of diseases like cholera, which often struck first and hardest in the poorer neighborhoods of towns or cities, both clergy and laypersons presented the argument that these outbreaks resulted from the intemperance or moral turpitude of the victims. After all, the arguments went, why else were so many of the initial victims from those lower classes of society? The media accounts of the outbreaks typically supported the argument with their observations that the victim was a drunkard, or of low moral character. No less a personage than George Templeton Strong, founder of the United States Sanitary Commission and a lawyer and noted diarist in New York, wrote that epidemics were most devastating among the lower classes since cholera "is God's judgment on the poor for neglecting His sanitary laws."[27]

The Irish were particularly singled out for judgment, building on the stereotype that this class of immigrants was the source of epidemic disease. Even before the potato famines of the 1840s, the Irish represented nearly half of all immigrants into the United States. While a significant number settled in New England, others migrated to New York or cities farther west, including Detroit. The large majority of these immigrants were poor and unskilled, with little choice but to live in those areas in which resources were often neglected. Little wonder that it was in this population that one would observe the judgment of "Divine Providence."

7

Between the Cholera "Wars"

As the city moved into the 1840s, the character of Detroit underwent a significant change. What had been a port city and trading center for travelers migrating into the hinterlands and beyond was evolving into a city similar in some ways to those in the East. Streets were lined with shops and businesses. As a more affluent class of citizens began to develop, tree-lined streets and more elaborate homes began to appear in what became residential neighborhoods. By 1840 the population had increased to approximately 9,000 persons, as more travelers decided to establish roots in the city; Detroit's population increased significantly as the 1840s proceeded, reaching 21,000 by the end of the decade. Though the occasional random case of cholera would appear—the disease had now become endemic throughout the western regions of the country— no large-scale outbreak would take place for some 15 years after the 1834 outbreak had subsided. Physicians would still remain ignorant of the infectious nature of the disease, but with improved sanitation and a cleaner water supply, water-borne diseases such as cholera remained in the background; other diseases such as influenza or typhoid fever, endemic in most cities of the period, would continue to present a challenge. Physicians remained busy in dealing with the diseases of the time, even if cholera was for a time no longer among them. For example, Detroit physician and former mayor Zina Pitcher provided a list of the most important diseases, and the month in which he was most likely to encounter them:

January: Puerperal fever, erysipelas, typhoid fever
February: Uterine phlebitis, erysipelas, typhoid fever
March: Erysipelas, typhoid fever, puerperal fever

April: Erysipelas, typhoid fever, puerperal fever
May: Puerperal fever, typhoid fever
June: Typhoid fever, dysentery
July: Dysentery, typhoid fever
August: Typhoid fever, dysentery, erysipelas
September: Dysentery, puerperal fever, erysipelas
October: Typhoid fever, dysentery, erysipelas
November: Typhoid fever, dysentery, erysipelas
December: Dysentery, typhoid fever, erysipelas, scarlet fever[1]

Erysipelas, a skin infection, and puerperal fever, often referred to as childbed fever, were the result of streptococcal infections. Puerperal fever in particular was a terrible disease that often afflicted women in the days following delivery. It was frequently transmitted on the hands of physicians, many of whom conducted their own autopsies on patients who had previously died — sometimes from puerperal fever itself — and who would move from patient to patient without hand washing. It is no surprise that erysipelas and puerperal fever (and scarlet fever as well) would be coincident with each other, given the same etiological agent is associated with each. Despite the twenty-first century knowledge of the central role played by infectious agents in disease, the medical staff in some hospitals must on occasion still be reminded to clean their hands prior to examining a patient.

Preventives or treatments for cholera continued to appear in the press, as physicians published their pet "cures." Sometimes they appeared to work, though in most of these instances one must question whether the patient was even suffering from cholera; dysentery and other diarrheal diseases were continuous problems, and though rarely fatal in adults, exhibited symptoms similar to those of cholera. Some of the recommendations provided to potential patients even made sense, as when citizens were advised to remove stagnant or standing water around their houses, and in particular to clean out any "dung heaps" and sewers. Persons were urged to avoid fresh fruit and raw or undercooked vegetables. Again, such precautions did make a modicum of sense, given that typhoid or cholera bacilli could be associated with such foods. It was also recommended that drinking water should be of "high quality."

If cholera did strike, patients should "wrap themselves in warm blankets, roll a swathe of warm flannel sprinkled with hot spirits of turpentine or whiskey, round the body, extending from the chest to hips, and take a teaspoonful of brandy or whiskey in a little water, with fifteen drops of laudanum, repeating it every hour, if the attack be not checked, until a third dose has been taken, but do not venture further in the use of laudanum without medical advice."[2] Some physicians took exception to the use of laudanum. Drs. John Ellis and S.B. Thayer, editors of the then-new publication *Michigan Journal of Homeopathy*, wrote in an editorial in response to the recommendation of laudanum:

> Gentlemen of the Board of Health, are you not yet satisfied with the use of opium in the treatment of diarrheas? For more than 3,000 years has this remedy and its preparations been used, in the treatment of these diseases, yet how generally do they fail to cure ... not less than one-half, or even two-thirds, have gone down to their graves, hurried onward by your opium ... with astringents and calomel thrown in.... In view of the probable appearance of the cholera in Detroit within the next few months, and of the fact, that from fifty to eighty out of every one hundred attacked die under every method of treating, this disease cannot be discovered.

As editors of a homeopathic journal, Ellis and Thayer had their own views as to proper treatment.

> We heartily agree with the many sanitary suggestions that have been made, and are being vigorously carried out by your body [Board of Health], for the thorough cleaning of the city, not only as it relates to Cholera, but to every other disease. But cleanliness alone, although it may mitigate the severity, never prevented the spread of smallpox or scarlet fever, or any other contagious or epidemic disease of a specific origin. [The concept of an infectious agent was of course unknown in 1848.] Such disease must be met by a specific capable of protecting the system against the influence of the noxious cause. The proper specific remedy is that which is capable of producing similar symptoms [i.e., a homeopathic remedy] in the healthy subject, to those of the disease we wish to guard him against. For instance: Smallpox is prevented by vaccination. Scarlet fever is prevented, or materially modified, by Belladonna, with certainty. Cuprum and Veratrum [copper and toxic herbs, respectively] are recommended as preventives of the Cholera, from the fact that they produce similar symptoms.[3]

Ellis and Thayer were correct in one respect when they predicted an epidemic of cholera was on the horizon, though the basis for that prediction is unclear. Cases had appeared that season both in St. Louis and New York City, though none were reported in Detroit itself. It is possible they were simply making an assumption of its appearance, albeit a correct one.

The *Michigan Journal of Homeopathy* was the first such medical journal to be published in the state. The November 1848 issue was among the first, and last, for the publication. The journal closed within a year.

Michigan Medical Society

The original medical society for the Territory of Michigan had been established by an act of the Legislative Council in June 1819. Physicians and surgeons within the territory were authorized to meet in Detroit, the largest town in the territory, in July of that year for the purpose of organizing a medical society. The same act authorized each county to likewise organize medical establishments, with the authority to test applicants wishing to practice medicine, and to grant diplomas, at a cost of $10, the diploma then being necessary to establish such a practice.[4] William Brown was elected president, Stephen Henry vice-president and Randall Rice treasurer. Requirements for becoming a physician were relatively simple considering the importance of the profession: two courses of lectures and an apprenticeship of three years working with a preceptor.

Among the early members of the society was Dr. William Beaumont, who in August 1826 provided an account to the society of his studies on gastric digestion observed through an open stomach wound of a patient on Mackinac Island; that presentation was described in an earlier chapter.

Meanwhile Detroit continued to grow, and the medical facilities that had proven inadequate during the 1834 outbreak had to be addressed. In addition, Michigan was officially admitted to the United States as the 26th state in January 1837. As a result the existing territorial medical society was no longer in existence. That year the first informal medical society in Detroit was organized. More a medical club than an official society, it was known as the Sydenham Medical Society of Detroit, named for the seventeenth century British physician Thomas Sydenham. Its founding members included Dr. Zina Pitcher, well respected for his work during the cholera epidemics, and Drs. George Russell and Adrian

7. Between the Cholera "Wars"

R. Terry, who were in partnership with each other. At that time the city of Detroit counted a mere several dozen trained physicians in the population of 9,000 persons.

The original Medical Society of Michigan was disbanded in 1844; most of its members lived in Detroit, and few issues were tackled that were considered significant beyond the city, anyway. There were also several controversies that had developed, mostly centered on how (or whether) to license someone to practice medicine. In 1846 a new medical society was formed, known as the Wayne County Medical Society. Its first president was Dr. Charles Ege. Ege had been graduated from the University of Pennsylvania Medical School, and at the time he came to Detroit in 1845 he had been assistant surgeon in the Philadelphia Alms House. Ege served as president until 1849. During the outbreak of cholera that year his wife was among the victims. Ege resigned and moved to California.

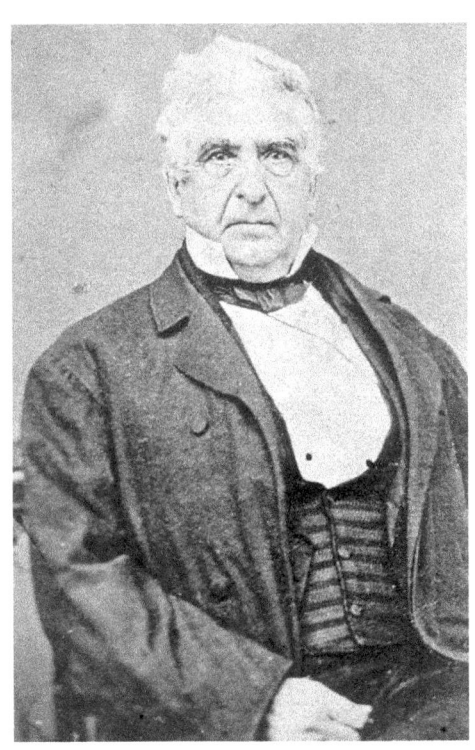

Zina Pitcher, twice mayor of Detroit (1840–1841, 1843), physician, botanist (image from the History of Medicine, National Library of Medicine).

Dr. Charles Tripler was elected vice-president of the society. Tripler had been graduated from medical school in 1838, and immediately enlisted in the army, where he served as a surgeon. He was posted at Fort Wayne in Detroit at the time of his membership in the society. Later during the Civil War, Triplett earned promotions to chief medical officer of the Department of the Ohio, eventually becoming a brevetted brigadier general.

Other officers in the society included Dr. Lucretius Cobb as secretary, Randall Rice as treasurer, and Drs. Peter Klein, Richard Inglis and A.L. Leland as censors. Additional members, many among the prominent physicians of the city, were Zina Pitcher, H.P. Cobb and Adrian Terry.[5]

Portions of the society's constitution immediately generated controversy, again over the question of licensing. Section 7 read: "The medical societies established as aforesaid may examine all students who shall present themselves for that purpose, and, if found qualified, may license them to practice as physicians, and give diplomas therefore ... to authorize the person obtaining the same to practice physic or surgery ... in any part of this state." Section 9 continued, "When any student shall have been examined or licensed by any county medical society, but shall in all cases make application thereafter to the State Medical Society, etc. Any license obtained contrary to the above was void." An example of such a license was the following, issued to one Edward Batwell: "Whereas, Edward Batwell hath exhibited unto us satisfactory testimony that he is entitled to a license to practice physic and surgery. Now know ye, that by virtue of the power and authority vested in us by law, we do grant unto said Edward Batwell the privilege of practicing physic and surgery in this state, together with all the rights and immunities which usually appertain to physicians."[6] The society therefore had the sole right to license prospective physicians based upon an oral examination, in effect disregarding any other qualifications, which might include medical training. And medical schools of the time were often that in name only, with students receiving minimal experience in anatomy—body snatching for such schools was a common vocation, given the paucity of such subjects—or in most other subjects standard in modern schools.

So what was the specific issue generating any controversy? What objection would be raised to the licensing of trained—however the term was applied—physicians? What objection was there for the study of medical subjects, including anatomy? The major difficulty, as noted above, was in the procurement of dead bodies. Unless a person willed their body for science, an uncommon occurrence, schools had no ready source of such study subjects. Consequently only the larger medical schools, mostly in the East, had any mechanism for the study of anatomy.

The other issue in contention was the question of the licensing practice itself. Should a person, by law, have such a license, or might they simply call themselves "doctor," start a practice, and let the buyer beware? The nineteenth century was one in which citizens had an

7. Between the Cholera "Wars"

extreme suspicion of anything that resembled government regulation; the term snake-oil salesman was well deserved through this period. Some felt that by allowing free competition, anyone attempting to practice would be subject to the marketplace. Only the best physicians would survive. Charles Darwin had yet to publish his theory, but natural selection was clearly at issue here.

In January 1844, Dr. Zina Pitcher submitted a petition to the state legislature requesting "a legalization" for the study of anatomy, primarily a means to obtain dead subjects for study, and the repeal of any laws affecting the study of medicine. The bill, discussed in the legislature that March, provided "that the bodies of all criminals who shall die in the state prison, if the friends do not claim the body, or the criminal have made no provision for his burial, and also the bodies of those who have been capitally executed [no longer applying by this time], shall be delivered over to a medical society."[7] The goal of the legislation was to provide a means to acquire such bodies for medical training.

The debate that took place in the state senate that same session addressed the issue of licensing, or for that matter whether any laws should be enacted that limited the ability of someone to practice. The marketplace should in effect decide. "Mr. Green ... believed that some regulations were necessary in order to protect the community against ignorant pretenders. The practice of medicine was of sufficient importance to demand the most severe and scrutinizing study. It was necessary that some guards should be set up to protect community." Mr. (Dr. Lewis) Starkey responded. In his opinion,

> It was useless to endeavor to legislate upon this subject; for the people would employ whom they pleased, whether quack or regular physicians. He believed that community would be more safe if the medical laws ... were repealed. The state of Pennsylvania had no laws whatever upon the subject of medicine, and there was not in the Union, perhaps in world, men of greater medical science than had lived in that state. By repealing that [restrictive] law we excited a laudable emulation among physicians. Each would strive to be more perfect in his profession. In the state of New York, where the medical laws were very stringent, the only exertion made was to pass an examination, and obtain a certificate, without conceiving it necessary to do anything more. By giving any person employed as a physician the power of collecting pay for his services, we also diminished the employment of quacks; for when persons found that their services had got to be paid for at any rate, they would employ those whom they thought would do best."

Others argued in a similar vein: "There were quacks in every profession, and as every person had a right to employ whom they pleased, the legislature should not pass a law prohibiting them from so doing.... If a man was killed by a quack, his estate should pay for it. This was the most effectual means of preventing their employment."[8] Politicians being politicians, then as well as now, regulation remained minimal.

Despite revisions in its statutes that might provide greater credibility to its members as practicing physicians, the 1846 version of the medical society lasted fewer than five years. Again the issue was "quackery," and who could be considered a physician. When a student appeared before the committee and passed the examination, he — and in these years only a "he" — received an impressive-looking certificate with a seal of authority attached, a paper with melted wax and an imprint of an eagle. However, the legislature continued to refuse the approval of any significant restrictions placed upon someone wishing to practice medicine; as argued years earlier and summarized above, the absence of regulation opened the door to quackery. Without regulation examinations became meaningless, which meant the medical society as a screening organization was likewise useless. In May 1851 the society was dissolved, saying, "This body, by the refusal of all law on the subject of their profession, are led to the conclusion that the public, ... from the signature to petitions addressed to the legislature on this subject, arrived at the belief that all wisdom and power are centered in them, rather than in those who have made medicine a study."[9]

The position of the existing society was not helped by the indifference demonstrated by other county societies: "Notice was given through the press, of the time and place of meeting. None of the members residing out of the city came to the annual session. None of the Presidents of County Medical Societies, who are ex-officio members of the State Society, came forward to take part in its proceedings. The object of this article is to awaken an interest in the medical men of the State, which shall prompt them to assist in giving life and efficiency to this society."[10] Despite the official name of Michigan Medical Society, members all resided in Detroit. County societies had their own parochial issues, and minimal interest in dealing with those problems confined largely to the city. Outside interest continued to remain minimal, and without any cooperation from the state legislature, the Michigan Medical Society would remain dissolved until 1853.

7. Between the Cholera "Wars"

The controversies associated with licensing of physicians were not unique either to Detroit or to Michigan in general. Licensing of physicians had been commonplace in most states until the 1830s, after which the stigma of "elitism" as applied to the practice of medicine opened the door to a more "democratic" view of the practitioner. During that period, as we have seen for Michigan, licensing laws were either eliminated, or so watered down that they became irrelevant. The situation as developed in Massachusetts during these years is a prime example. In 1818 and 1819 it was established that "no person, entering the practice of physic or surgery, shall be entitled to the benefit of law for the recovery of any debt or fee for professional services, unless he shall, previously to rendering these services, have been licensed by the officers of the Massachusetts Medical Society, or have been graduated a doctor of medicine in Harvard University." The requirements were eliminated in 1836, with the implication, as interpreted by the Massachusetts Sanitary Commission, being that "no restriction is laid upon anyone in the practice of physic, or in dealing in drugs or medicines. Anyone, male or female, learned or ignorant, an honest man or a knave, can assume the name of a physician, and 'practice' upon anyone, to cure or to kill, as either may happen, without accountability. 'It's a free country!'"[11]

The practice of medicine during this era was of course a male preserve; even having women serve as attendants was controversial, and would continue so until the Civil War. Still, there were stirrings on the issue of women being trained as physicians, at least back East:

> A Philadelphia letter writer, states that the female medical college [known as Female Medical College at its founding] in the city is progressing as satisfactorily as any friend of the rights of women could possibly desire; and all that is now wanted to complete the good work is the establishment of a Female Theological Seminary and a Female Law School. If women from the force of circumstances, must work for a livelihood, why should they be debarred from the liberal professions, and compelled to dwell among pots, or to make beds, or to measure out calico, or to work in factories, or to cook, wash scrub, darn and sew? Blessings on Miss [Elizabeth] Blackwell [first woman to receive a medical degree in the United States] for the practical idea; a social revolution is about to take place. In less than three years, something less than three hundred lovely and lovable girls, with straw bonnets, low neck dresses, gaiter boots, (if the fashions don't change in the meantime,) will be driving about the streets of Philadelphia in their gigs, killing and curing, according to the good old orthodox and allopathic system. Woman,

lovely woman, is the only proper attendant for the sick room; and if we are to be bled or physicked to death, let it be done with sweet smiles and gentle hands. With a young, blooming, blushing female physician to feel your pulse with her round tapering fingers, or to put her warm, soft, plump hand on your aching head, who wouldn't be sick? The danger is that Philadelphia will become frightfully unhealthy the moment these bewitching spinsters matriculate.[12]

The writer expressed the prejudices of the time, of course. Women in growing numbers would continue to join the health professions, though the areas in which they were able to practice would be limited for generations.

Detroit Sanitation

As recounted earlier, construction of the Grand Sewer was authorized by the Common Council in 1836 as a means to divert water directly into the Detroit River at Third Street. If drain water from rain had been the only liquid flowing through the sewer, there might not have been any problems. However, with the absence of any process of sewage treatment, a common situation of the time, raw sewage from residential or business sites routinely entered the stream, and ultimately passed into the Detroit River. Besides the obvious odors associated with the practice (and such smells were so ubiquitous that they were generally ignored until they became too obnoxious), any infectious agents present in the sewage would eventually mix with water used for eating or drinking.

The prevailing thinking was twofold. Nobody of course would want any hint of sewage in their drinking water. But intake pipes for such water were usually extended far out into the river, beyond the sites at which sewage entered the river. Second, to apply a modern phrase, "the solution to pollution was dilution"; it was felt water could purify itself, either by flowing out to the larger lake, or, in early twentieth century reasoning, through the growth of microbiota capable of breaking down impurities. Neither would apply to sanitation procedures of the 1840s.

The increase in population meant the old water reservoir constructed nearly a decade earlier was now obsolete. A new brick reservoir was constructed during 1837 and 1838. The new pumping system, known as the New Hydraulic Works, came into service in 1841 to supply water for the Fort Street reservoir; it was replaced a year later by a new iron reservoir.[13] The system still proved inadequate for the increase in population, doubling in size between 1840 and 1850. Engines for the reservoir pumped 24 hours a day; leakage compounded the problems. In 1849 a new, larger engine and pump were installed, as well as another new reservoir, located near today's Eastern Market site. By that year the system contained over four miles of iron mains supplemented by the older 35 miles of wooden mains. None of this addressed the problem of sewage contamination from the river. Once cholera again appeared in the city, it became inevitable that it would spread through the population.

The Presence of Cholera and Related Events: 1835–1850

Detroit was not unique among American cities during this period in being spared any large-scale outbreaks of the disease. The occasional ship docking in New York would have some passengers suffering from cholera, but even these were relatively few. Meanwhile cholera continued to rage in other portions of the world.

So how might one explain the disappearance of the disease during these 15 years or so after 1834? One simple explanation sometimes suggested was that those countries with which the United States was interacting were themselves largely free of the disease.[14] Is this explanation valid? England and Ireland make prime examples. The potato famine that began mid-decade in Ireland, exacerbating the grinding poverty, and the religious and ethnic discrimination by the English, forced a terrible choice upon the citizenry: either emigrate or starve. Nearly one million persons migrated to Canada or the United States, many settling on the East Coast. Many of the Irish also immigrated to the industrial cities of England — Liverpool or Glasgow — where they could not escape discrimination but at least could find a semblance of work. The politicians of England paid particular concern to what they perceived was an "inundation" of the Irish poor fleeing starvation, not just into port cities such as Liverpool, but in most of the larger cities of Great Britain. But it was through Liverpool that most of the immigrants passed, nearly 300,000 of them in 1847 alone; nearly half remained, either because they attempted to find jobs there, or because they simply had no money to travel any further. The port of Liverpool represented a staging point for immigrants originating in much of Europe — Chinese, Germans, some of whom would later carry cholera along with other trappings, and even Americans; Liverpool was also infamous for the number of whorehouses established to "service" the well-heeled among those passing through, an estimation of over 700.[15]

But it was the Irish immigrants who created the greatest concern. They often carried disease with them, typhoid certainly, and something pejoratively referred to as Irish fever, likely typhus. In 1847, Liverpool, a city of some 250,000 persons, reported 100,000 cases of diarrhea, much of it being dysentery, and over 60,000 cases of assorted fevers.[16] Nevertheless, cholera was not among those diseases the Irish brought with them during these first years of the famine. The period of the early to mid–1840s in England in fact was one of declining epidemics. Various explanations attempt to explain why, the most common being that the improved living conditions among those who had jobs reduced exposure to illness. But this disappearance of epidemic disease could only be applied to cholera; other water-borne diseases such as typhoid or dysentery remained common.[17] A more likely explanation was that neither the English nor the Irish, isolated on their islands, were being exposed to the disease during these years. And the English and Irish represented well over half of the immigrants to the United States during this same period. A substantial number of German immigrants also arrived in the United States during the 1840s, but as was true for England, cholera did not appear in significant numbers in the German states until nearly the end of the decade. So the simplest explanation may indeed be the best. Unlike the outbreak of the disease back in 1832, which was brought to Canada from Ireland, cholera did not appear in the United States until 1849 because it was not epidemic in western Europe during this period.

The situation changed drastically for western Europe, including England, by the latter years of the decade. Cholera of course had never disappeared; it remained endemic in the same places in which previous outbreaks had taken place: India, Afghanistan and other regions in that portion of the world. Britain again became one of the conduits through which the disease began to spread. British troops became exposed in India, and by 1840 brought the disease with them to China, where some were subsequently stationed. From there trade routes carried the disease into Russia, and from there towards Europe. At the same time cholera moved west on shipping and migration routes into the Saudi peninsula. Cholera killed over 15,000 pilgrims in Mecca in 1846, and from there moved into both Egypt and portions of eastern Europe. By 1848 the disease had returned to England, again carried on trading ships originating from portions of Europe in which cholera had by now reappeared. It was this outbreak in London that the English physician John Snow traced to a contaminated water supply provided by one of the major suppliers to the city, Southwark and Vauxhall. The lower portion of the Thames River, the source of the water, had been contaminated by effluent from a ship that had previously docked in Hamburg at the time a cholera outbreak was taking place; the story of John Snow is presented in a later chapter. Over 14,000 persons died from the disease in London alone that year. However, even before Snow's epidemiological studies on the source of the cholera, suspicion began to focus during these years on water as the source. For example, a public notice for the "Liberty of Havering-Atte-Bower," an administrative area now part of London, warned the public as to methods of avoiding the illness: "To guard against accumulations of refuse matter in drains, cess-pools, dust-bins, and dirt-heaps, and to purify such receptacles by solution of Chloride of Lime. To maintain in a cleanly and wholesome condition all reservoirs, cisterns and sinks, and to allow impurities, where practical, to be carried away by running water."[18] The magistrate who published the warning would not have been aware of the mechanism by which standing water would have carried the disease. Even so, he had correctly linked exposure to impure water as possibly playing a role in spread of the disease.

Meanwhile cholera jumped from England to Ireland late in 1848, at a time in which significantly increased immigration to the United States and Canada was taking place. Between 1846 and 1850, the peak years of the potato famine, an average of 200,000 Irish entered the United States each year, while an additional 100,000 migrated to Canada.

Canadians, as citizens of the British Empire, were particularly concerned about the Irish now coming to North America. England had always encouraged some emigration to Canada, somehow reasoning that while this would help solve the Irish "problem," it would also encourage the Irish to remain associated with the mother country. Fares to Canada were significantly cheaper than those to the United States. Of course this would not stop a family from first entering Canada, and then traveling south to the United States. But things changed in the mid–1840s. Traditional Irish immigrants to Canada had been members of what was considered a higher social class: merchants or successful farmers. As a result of the famine, combined with British practices towards the island, the immigrants in the latter half of the decade were considered "low Irish," depicted in the stereotype as dirty and malodorous. Canadians remembered how cholera was brought to North America in 1832, primarily among the Irish immigrants to Montreal and Quebec.[19] And as we have seen, from there cholera moved across the border into Buffalo, beginning an epidemic that claimed thousands. The newer concerns subsequently proved justified. Some of the immigrants in 1848 and 1849 carried cholera with them, likely those disembarking in New York. Only a few were infected, but there were enough to reintroduce the disease.

8

The Epidemic of 1849

For 15 years the United States had been fortunate in that cholera made no inroads on American shores. The population of Detroit had doubled during the decade of the 1840s, reaching some 21,000 individuals. The situation changed rapidly as 1848 came to a close. Citizens of both New York and New Orleans, likely about the same time, became exposed to cholera as passengers on arriving ships carried the disease with them. Every steamboat arriving in New Orleans by now was considered a floating pest-house. From New Orleans the disease spread west into Texas and north along the Mississippi.[1]

Both New Orleans and New York could be considered the focal points for the epidemic, which would subsequently reach Detroit by May of 1849. That the island of Manhattan successfully avoided an outbreak during the winter months and early spring was primarily due to the cold weather, which limited movement among its population; however, the weather did not prevent the disease from reaching the shores of the city. On November 9, 1848, the ship *New York* left the French port of Le Havre, ostensibly cholera free. The French port had apparently been spared the disease, but many of the passengers had embarked from German cities where cholera was already present. Two weeks into the voyage trunks were opened on the ship, which contained the clothes of earlier victims of cholera. Whether this was the source of the infection on board the ship, or whether someone had already been infected when the ship sailed, is open to conjecture. The short incubation period associated with cholera might suggest the former, not that it really mattered once the disease had appeared. Regardless of its source, by the time the ship arrived in New York harbor seven passengers had already died, and another 11 were sick with the disease.[2] The appearance of cholera was reported in newspapers:

> On Friday morning the packet ship *New York* ... arrived and anchored in the bay, nearly midway between Staten and Long Island, having lost seven persons by death of Asiatic Cholera — When the ship left Havre, the place, the crew and passengers were perfectly healthy, and the passengers continued so about fifteen days, when the sickness took place, in the steerage, among the passengers there. On Saturday [November 16], several sick persons were landed at the Quarantine [located on Staten island], and on Sunday morning two died of the disease. On Sunday all the steerage passengers, about 325 in number, were taken from the ship on board the steamboat *Sampson* to the United States stores, within the hospital walls, and are all housed in those buildings. There are several persons sick, and one is reported to have died this morning. The cabin passengers have all come up to the city, and so has the steamboat *Sampson*, that took out the passengers. Thus the communication between the infected ship and the city has been uninterrupted.... All the physicians on Staten Island, the Health Officers included, that have seen the present cases, pronounce them of a mild character, and most of them have yielded readily to mild treatment.[3]

To what was the outbreak attributed? It was suggested that as the ship approached the shores of America it encountered unusually warm weather for November, which according to the authorities may have triggered the disease. The New York Board of Health recommended that excessive eating and drinking should be avoided, and recommended as well as to avoid eating raw vegetables. If symptoms of the disease appeared, and no medical assistance was available, 15 to 20 drops of laudanum were recommended.[4]

The quarantine of the passengers had the desired effect, despite the assumption that those not confined to steerage, the cabin passengers, had avoided the disease. The outbreak was limited to those on the ship and did not immediately spread beyond Staten Island. However, the presence of cholera in New York was noted as far away as Detroit, and a prescient warning appeared in the local newspaper:

> Among all the interesting and exciting topics which now occupy the attention of the public, no one deserves more immediate notice from us who stay at home, than the expected invasion of cholera. That it will come is almost certain, and there is too much reason to think, that if it does come, it will give us fearful evidence of its power. A great proportion of our present population has come here since the former epidemic [1834], and many are, perhaps, not aware of the virulence with which it raged, and the devastation with which caused. There is no good reason to suppose that another epidemic would be less violent, and the great increase of our population will of course furnish

more victims.... Experience has shown that all quarantine regulations are ineffectual in stopping its march, it is emphatically 'the pestilence that walketh in darkness,' it has overstepped all natural boundaries, crossed mountains and seas, and set at naught all human precautions against its access.[5]

Dramatic? Perhaps. But the writer was correct. Conditions had significantly changed in the ensuing years since the previous outbreak. The size of susceptible populations had increased, not just in New York or Detroit, but in most American cities. Modes of transportation had become faster and more efficient. Whereas in 1834 most long-distance transportation involved relatively slow boats or ships, railroads were now making their appearance. A person exposed to cholera in New York or New Orleans could be hundreds of miles farther inland by the time symptoms first appeared, as seen in these cases:

> I hasten to inform you that the *General Lafayette* [steamboat] arrived here early this morning, having left New Orleans on the evening of the 29th [December]. No deaths of cholera on board — eleven cases cured. The clerk of the *Lafayette* reports 214 deaths at New Orleans on the 29th. She passed a flatboat loaded with ploughs from Maysville, Kentucky, near Helena, with three of the crew dead.... Two deaths on the *E.W. Stephens* from Memphis.... Six or seven cases of cholera in Memphis — bad along the coast. The Lafayette brought up about 100 passengers.[6]

The disease, which first appeared in New Orleans in the beginning of December, appeared in Memphis two weeks later, and in St. Louis a week after that, and Cincinnati by Christmas. By May the disease had spread throughout the trans–Mississippi region.[7] Among the victims who were likely exposed while visiting New Orleans that spring was ex-president James Polk, who died of cholera in June 1849, and Major-General William Worth, who had been among the commanders of the American army in the recent Mexican-American War. Worth died of the disease in May 1849 in San Antonio, where he had been sent by the war department. The city of Fort Worth was named in his honor.

The appearance of cholera in both New Orleans and New York in December, even if the disease had not yet given evidence of spreading to Detroit, resulted in the Common Council of Detroit re-establishing a Board of Health. Among the first actions of the board was an attempt to allay the fears of the general public, in part by providing a series of recommendations as to how to avoid exposure to the disease:

Through the Medical Journals of the day, we have had access to the recorded proceedings of Sanitary bodies, organized in view of the presence or approach of the cholera, not only in our own country, but in Europe. In these, we find the opinions of men eminent for ability, as to the nature, means of prevention and method of cure of this disease, based upon observations made during its former march over the old and new world, tested in some instances during its present incursion. We have found so much in these records that coincides with our own experience in the years 1832, 1833 and 1834, during its prevalence in the United States, that we have copied from the sources what seemed best adapted to the conditions of things, both present and prospective, in Detroit. [We present] the following summary of opinions or conclusions and recommendations: 1. The cholera, although propagated by a peculiar infection or morbitic poison, is not in a pure atmosphere communicated by the sick to their attendants. The dread of contagion, therefore, should not occasion friends to desert their sick or bury the dead with indecent haste. [The board was correct in that the contagion is not transmitted through the air. It could, however, be transmitted through contamination by fecal material.] 2. Sanitary arrangements, and not quarantine restrictions, constitute the best safeguards to the public health. [Though it is highly unlikely the board was aware of John Snow's studies taking place in London that year, which demonstrated the role of contaminated water, they were correct in attributing the spread to improper sanitation.] 3. The cholera is almost always, in this country, manifest by a premonitory diarrhea. This is its *first and curable stage* [italics in original]. At this time appropriate remedies will ward off an attack. If neglected or improperly treated, the stage of collapse supervenes, which in most cases, proves fatal. [Correct, though their mistake was in the method of proper intervention — which should be immediate rehydration.] 4. In persons of sound constitutions and good habits, few diseases are so easily averted, when the first warning symptoms of its attack are timely attended to and properly treated. It can be prevented in 80 or 90 of 100 cases, and here we would take occasion to warn the public not to use medicines as unduly as prophylactics [in the context of preventing disease, not the modern context of pregnancy] or preventives — for whatever is active enough to do good when required, must of course do harm if needlessly taken or administered. [Cholera was not the only illness characterized by diarrhea. Apparent "cures" often attributed to various methods of treatment likely were associated with other, milder, diarrheas.] 5. Observations and experience have shown, that certain conditions favor, in a special manner, the prevalence and mortality of cholera. These conditions are — low, damp situations, and rich alluvial soils, wharves, banks of rivers and streams, moisture or dampness from any cause; collection of filth, of vegetable and animal matters, and whatever produces offensive and noxious effluvia and miasma; foul and impure atmosphere, proceeding from imperfect ventilation, uncovered drains, narrow courts and alleys, crowded densely with inhabitants,

8. The Epidemic of 1849

and in fine, whatever tends, either morally or physically to depress the forces of life or disorder the system in any manner.

As to how to avoid the illness:

> From the nature of the complaint, it is evident that much depends upon keeping the body warm. Flannel next the skin should be a universal article of apparel ... the diet should be particularly attended to.... All crude and raw vegetables, as well as violent and purgative medicines, are calculated to do mischief.... The preservation of a calm and composed state of mind is all important, and may do more than is generally supposed, in preventing the onset of the disease. It is the result of experience, that all epidemics are aggravated more or less by mental disturbance, whether in the shape of actual panic or low despondency. To the cholera, this is particularly applicable.... With regard to the treatment of cholera, it should be observed that, as a general rule, the disease does not attack so suddenly as to preclude the possibility of calling in timely medical assistance. A relaxed state of the bowels for a longer or shorter period, gives notice of its approach.... When professional aid cannot be obtained immediately, and where simple relaxation of the bowels exists, 15 or 20 drops of laudanum may be taken, to be repeated in one or two hours, according to circumstances.... When the symptoms are more severe, and the patient is cold, in addition to the laudanum, he should be put immediately to bed, between blankets, add every appliance in the shape of bottles of hot water, bags of hot salt or sand, frictions, etc. be diligently resorted to. A strong mustard poultice, too, should be applied over the region of the stomach, to remain on until it produces smarting of the skin. In addition to this, a little brandy and water should be given, with the view of restoring warmth.[8]

Of course little in the way of palliative treatment — warmth, some laudanum and a little brandy and water — would do much beyond making the patient a little more comfortable.

Meanwhile, in New York, health authorities had hoped the quarantine of the *New York*'s passengers on Staten Island would prevent the spread of the disease to the mainland. During the weeks of December and early January in which the outbreak had been taking place, over 60 of the passengers had become ill, with about half dying from the disease. In the 10 to 15 years since the previous epidemic, little had been accomplished by the authorities of the city to deal with any potential appearance of the disease, and the lack of preparation included a failure to build any form of sanitary facility to house any victims. It was even unclear where such facilities would be placed. Suddenly hundreds of persons were to be placed in quarantine, with no proper means of caring for these individuals. Customs warehouses on the island were quickly converted into barracks and hospital wards. But with too few officers to oversee too many people, few of whom had any desire to remain in the presence of cholera victims, scores of persons began "eloping," scaling the walls and making their way across the water to Manhattan or New Jersey; some carried the disease with them.[9] Not surprisingly, sporadic cases of cholera appeared in the poorest areas of the city, generally the most crowded portions of New York. As long as the winter weather remained, those cases had few opportunities to spread from what were looming as focal points of infection. But things began to change in the spring. Among the most destitute places in the city was the area known as Five Points, an area of lower Manhattan in which there was an intersection of five streets. During the mid–nineteenth century the neighborhood, predominantly inhabited by poor Irish, was among the most notorious in the city. It was here that the 1849 cholera outbreak in New York likely began.

On May 15 and 16 at least four deaths from cholera were reported in a lodging house on Orange Street in the Five Points area.[10] There was not a single cholera hospital in the city at the beginning of the outbreak, and even weeks later only the second floor of a tavern and a few public schools served as makeshift hospitals in the emergency. Following the report of cholera in the Five Points neighborhood on the 16th, a Sanatory (sic) Committee was established through the city board of health, the job of which was to maintain a daily monitoring of the disease. Additional recommendations forbade the sale of fruits and vegetables from the ubiquitous pushcarts, and required owners of tenements to clean their properties.[11] How quickly tenement owners responded to the request is unknown, but one may surmise they did no more than was necessary. New Yorkers responded either by fleeing the city, in some instances carrying the disease with them, or by turning again to religion. And while the disease did not spread as rapidly as it had during the previous outbreaks in the 1830s — the water source had been made significantly safer during the interim — by the time the epidemic in New York had ended in the fall, over 5,000 persons had died from the disease.

From exactly which direction cholera began its approach to Detroit — west from New York City or Buffalo, or north by way of the Mississippi and its tributaries — is unclear. It may very well have been coming from both directions. During March and April alone, over 1,000

8. The Epidemic of 1849

deaths in New Orleans were attributed to cholera. One could follow cholera's progression during the spring of 1849 by the towns that reported its appearance: From Louisville, Kentucky the third week of March, "the steamer *Bride*, from New Orleans, passed up the river on Saturday night [March 24]. During the trip there were ten deaths from cholera on board.... Four persons were buried at the mouth of Salt River. From Tuesday the [March] 13th to Monday the 19th, 27 deaths have occurred among the troops now stationed at Jefferson Barracks [St. Louis]. Our informant states that the fatal disease in all its symptoms was that of cholera. During the week ending Monday last [26th], there were ninety-four deaths in the city of St. Louis, twenty-four of which were children of the age of five years and younger. Of this number twenty-six are reported as having died of cholera."[12] By early May, if not sooner, cholera had reached Chicago by way of St. Louis: "Passengers that came over from Chicago ... report several cases of the cholera as having occurred in that city.... If the report is true, the cases have, no doubt, occurred among passengers who have arrived by the Illinois Canal from St. Louis, and the cities on the Mississippi."[13] Various towns in upper New York State reported sporadic cases as well, including the port city of Buffalo. The appearance in Buffalo began with a steamship originating at Chicago. The ship traveled north on Lake Michigan past Mackinac Island and south through the lakes, eventually working its way to Buffalo where it arrived May 13, about the same time the outbreak was beginning in New York City. Additional steamboats coming from Chicago and Cincinnati that arrived in Buffalo in June carried passengers with the disease. By the end of that summer over 3,000 cases of cholera would spread through Buffalo, with nearly one-third of the victims dying from the disease. Since there was regular steamship traffic between Buffalo and Detroit, any passengers infected with cholera could quickly carry it to the latter city. Aware of the danger, at least some officials in Detroit as early as May 14 recommended the city quarantine any passengers arriving from Buffalo.

As in previous epidemics, there was no shortage of ideas as to how to protect oneself from the disease. Among the newer "prescriptions" was this:

> During the year 1832 when we were first visited with the cholera, I learned from some source, that the spirits of camphor, taken in small doses, was a certain specific. Being at the time connected with the Post Office in this city

> [Detroit] I procured several dozen of small phials, which I filled with small spirits of camphor, and gave one to each of the clerks and letter carriers, with directions whenever they felt any premonitory symptoms of the cholera, to take ten drops in a tablespoon of water, and if that did not relieve them, to repeat the dose every fifteen minutes until they found relief. Neither the clerks nor any of the carriers had the cholera, although the latter were constantly exposed by visiting every part of the city in the discharge of their duty.
>
> Two persons in my own family were attacked with cholera, one of them severely, to whom I administered camphor before any physician arrived, and they were both cured.[14]

Since camphor is occasionally used as a food additive, one can at least concede the treatment would do no harm. Nor is the aroma of camphor repulsive, at least if one likes mothballs.

Camphor was among the homeopathic prophylactic procedures practiced at the time. If the patient was unable to swallow any liquid that contained the ingredient, camphor could be applied to a cloth, which could then be placed on the face of the patient. Patients were also warned not to use camphor in large quantities, as it could counteract the efficacy of other recommended medications such as veratrum (herbs) or cuprum (copper).

So who would be most subject to an attack by cholera? There were the usual suspects, of course, the poor or the intemperate. This time an additional risk factor was added to those most prone to infection: "Dr. A.G. Goodler, late surgeon U.S. Infantry, in giving an abstract of his theory and practice of the cholera, in a communication addressed to the President, says, we find the Negro more subject to it than the white man, the white man more than the white woman. The reason he gives for the selection is, the Negro has more nitrogen and less oxygen about his person than the white man. It is this superabundance of nitrogen which he considers to be allied to the remote cause of cholera."[15] Besides the obvious racial overtone, one must wonder where or when he carried out such empirical studies.

Whether or not Goodler's theory produced any following is unknown. No similar references to a racial bias in the disease were printed. But this represented one example of the growing frustrations found in populations at risk, willing to accept almost any hypothesis dealing with the cause of the disease, or a preventive or treatment. Physi-

8. The Epidemic of 1849

cians seemed to accept almost any outlandish idea if it seemed to explain the origin and spread of the disease. Even the wind itself could be at fault, with a measure of prejudice added for flavor:

> We believe and aver, that the predisposing cause of cholera is simply and nothing else, but the pestilential breath of the ever tormented and ever tormenting "wandering Jew" who for some unknown cause, periodically circumnavigates this planet. His approach may be always anticipated by the prevalence of a strong steady current of wind blowing from the east towards the west, which is so piercing, withering, and repulsive, not only to all animals, but vegetables also, that they wither and die, if continued for a long or uninterrupted period of time, of from twenty-five to thirty days. Nor is this a novel doctrine. All sacred and profane history from the earliest stages of the world, both unite in handing down to us the fact that the east wind from time immemorial, blew mildew, pestilence and famine.... All the medical officers who have written upon the laws of life, disease and its causes, of the least celebrity, since the days of Paraselsus [a fifteenth century German physician], but have indicated the principle that all the diseases that the flesh is heir to, are always heightened and increased on the prevalence of an eastern wind, and ameliorated immediately on a change of an opposite direction.... Cholera never has made its appearance in this or any other country, without the wind has blown directly from the east for the period of twenty-five to thirty days.
>
> Why is the east wind a predisposing cause to produce cholera? It is simply because, that the good health of the system depends upon an equilibrium of action between the surface and the centre of the body, that the east wind repels the heat and fluids of the body from the surface towards the centre, and an opposite wind from the centre to the circumference, that the stomach and bowels being encroached upon by this means for a long time, and thus predisposed, on adding other exciting causes as mentioned before, is induced.
>
> The east wind, before cholera made its 1832 appearance in New York, blew uninterruptedly for the period of thirty-two days. It has blown from the east for the last two months here, for fifteen and twenty days without an interruption of but twenty-four hours.
>
> What are the best remedies? I answer, those that will counteract, and maintain the current of warmth of the system from the centre to the circumference, and thereby continue the equilibrium of health.
>
> It is this that makes the Chicago pill, of Charcoal and Sulpher [sic], a good pill, from its maintaining a current from the centre to the surface. Sulpher will act on the pores so as to blacken silver in the pocket in twenty-four hours; but this pill may be combined with other remedies better than that is yet.[16]

Charcoal and sulphur were among the common medications sometimes classified as "Western medicines," medications developed by pioneers in the absence of trained doctors—not that such individuals even if they had been present had more than a superficial knowledge of disease—and often based upon folk remedies either from the old country, or learned from interactions with Native Americans. Sulphur pills and sulphur candies were particularly popular during the 1840s and 1850s for treatment of cholera. That spring of 1849 one Dr. J.H. Byrd managed to provide a scientific explanation for the (alleged) effectiveness of sulphur pills. Byrd happened upon an article authored by a German chemist, Dr. Christian Schönbein, discoverer of ozone, which suggested that the presence of influenza was the result of changes in the ozone concentration in the atmosphere. By chemically analyzing the concentration of ozone, advocates of ozone therapy found a correlation between increased levels of the ozone molecule in the atmosphere and the severity of influenza outbreaks. Since cholera epidemics seemed to follow those of influenza outbreaks, it followed in Byrd's mind that the cause of both epidemics, an increase in ozone levels, was the same. So the question became how does one reduce either the levels of ozone, or at least neutralize its effects? It was believed that cholera never broke out in regions with sulphur springs. Hence sulphur would appear to be the neutralizing agent. Assuming the reduced incidence of cholera at these sites was real, the explanation that sulphur might inactivate or kill the actual infectious agent is not one that would have been explored in the 1840s.

Byrd had been bothered by stomach cramps and diarrhea, symptoms, he felt, of cholera. He and several friends exhibiting similar digestive problems ingested several grains of sulphur, and the symptoms disappeared. The same procedure was tried on others exhibiting similar symptoms, and within hours all symptoms of cholera had been ameliorated.[17] By mid-summer sulphur pills were available throughout much of the country. Even more extreme measures were popular during these years, not even including those endorsing morphine or ether. Physicians had recommended strychnine, tobacco-smoke enemas and even immersion in ice water.[18] Calomel—mercury—still remained popular with some physicians who were willing to overlook its side effects. Patients became increasingly unwilling to subject themselves to such treatments, and some physicians who continued to prescribe it often found themselves without patients. One side effect was considered a positive trait: the bleeding of gums signified the calomel was having an effect.

8. The Epidemic of 1849

Despite increasing evidence to the contrary, whether to prevent episodes of panic similar to those which had taken place 15 years earlier, or simply to protect business interests, the local media in Detroit preferred to deny that any such outbreak was taking place:

> We understand stories are in circulation in the interior that the cholera is raging in this city! In conversation with a farmer yesterday, he informed us that he was warned against coming to the city with his produce, as 20 per day were dying with the cholera here. Another told us that he was told the city was very unhealthy, and he would be unable to sell any produce, as business was at a standstill.
>
> Now, we would inform our readers that *not a single case of cholera* [italics in original] has been known to exist in the city — that Detroit was never so healthy as this very day. A physician informed us yesterday, that in a twelve years practice he had never known so little sickness. So far as business is concerned, we would inform our friends that it is quite brisk. If our merchants and others do not pay as high prices for wool and produce as it is worth, don't sell to them. They will then be forced to pay a good and fair price.[19]

Newspaper accounts of deaths during this period preferred euphemisms, if they recounted any deaths at all. In June, for example, 35 burials in the city were reported, none of the deaths being attributed to cholera. Two of the dead, however, succumbed to having "died from drinking cold water." It was not until July 2 that the first official notice of a death from cholera was acknowledged. Announcements were routinely made as to the total deaths (burials) during the summer months, but names were not provided, and rarely was any specific cause of death included. It was not until the epidemic had peaked that the local newspapers were forced to report the presence of cholera. For example, during the last week of July there were 33 burials in the city. Seven of the dead were then acknowledged as having died of the disease. The number of deaths became so large during these weeks that coffins were often transported on ordinary drays or sledges.[20] The complaint voiced by the farmer, as recounted above, became increasingly common as citizens expressed their fears that the numbers with which they were presented were completely inaccurate. They knew cholera was in the city, whether the authorities acknowledged it or not.

The Board of Health did what it could. The Common Council allocated $2,400 for cleaning of streets, filling of stagnant pools and providing care for those stricken. But disposal of sewage remained a significant problem. In the absence of rain, necessary to flush the sewers—albeit directly into the river—excretions originating in the privies, animal carcasses decomposing on the streets, or waste from slaughterhouses continued to accumulate; the odors at times in the summer were beyond description. In 1869 Dr. Samuel Duffield, professor of chemistry at Detroit Medical College, calculated an estimate of the quantity of material found in the sewers. Extrapolating his numbers to the 1849 population of Detroit, approximately 5,000 pounds of solid filth would enter the sewers every day, in addition to some 100,000 pounds of liquid waste daily. This did not even take into account other sources of contamination, including animal waste. What is surprising is not just that cholera had not become endemic, reappearing every year, but that other waterborne diseases were not even more common.[21]

Numbers released by the authorities, including the Board of Health, are conceded to have been artificially low:

> The whole number of fatal cases of cholera reported by the physicians was 73. The sextons report 159. [It is unclear whether these were overlapping numbers, or represent two separate sets of dead.] Of this number at least 30 were strangers left by boats. Many of the cases reported by the sextons, says the Committee [associated with the Board of Health], we are satisfied were not cholera. There being no attending physician, cases of sudden death were almost always attributed to that disease. The Committee thinks that the whole number of deaths by cholera does not exceed 120, of whom 30 were strangers, and 90 were citizens.[22]

The precise number of deaths in Detroit from cholera that summer, usually described as greater than 300, is at best an educated guess; the precise number will remain unknown. However, one can produce an estimate based upon the number of internments, numbers which were generally given space in the local newspapers. During July there were 781 reported internments. For the first three weeks during the month of August, 280 deaths were reported, a total of greater than 1,000 during the peak months of the epidemic. If one uses as precedence the proportion of total deaths from cholera in Detroit during the 1854 epidemic in which more than 50 percent of deaths during the epidemic were attributed to cholera, it is likely the estimate of 300 deaths during the 1849 outbreak is a minimum figure.

9

Epidemic of 1854

Cholera may have disappeared from Detroit during the interval between 1849 and 1854, but it was certainly present elsewhere in the Midwest. Chicago reported over 600 deaths from cholera in 1852, and outbreaks were reported in other Western cities such as St. Louis. The disease was still in epidemic form in much of Europe during these years as well, and no less than 28 ships were allegedly carrying passengers with the disease to American ports; over 1,100 deaths attributed to cholera were reported on these voyages.[1] Ships carrying passengers ill with the disease arrived in New Orleans beginning late in 1853 and continuing into the early winter months of 1854. Nevertheless it was several months before the disease broke out in that city. Once that epidemic did begin to take place, the disease quickly spread north, followed the Mississippi River as it had five years earlier, and appeared in port cities along the way such as St. Louis and Memphis. The first cases of cholera that broke out in Chicago were reported in April. Over 3,500 deaths due to cholera were reported in St. Louis that summer, the largest number of such victims reported by any city, while some 1,400 deaths were reported in Chicago before the epidemic ran its course. In attempts to limit the outbreaks, beginning in the spring authorities in New Orleans refused embarkation of passengers. In addition to providing little in the way of protection to the citizens of New Orleans, this practice served merely to send the disease farther upriver.

The first cases reported in New York appeared in June of that year, actually preceding the outbreak in Detroit. However, dates in this case may be misleading. Ships carrying passengers from Europe with cholera arrived in that East Coast port city as early as November 1853. Many of these immigrants were sent onward in their travels, carrying baggage that may also have been contaminated with the cholera agent. Other ships disembarked passengers into the city who were clearly carrying the disease. On May 16 the ship *North America* arrived from Liverpool carrying 768 passengers, 17 of whom had died from cholera while in transit; among the remaining passengers, who were immediately placed in quarantine, 120 persons developed cholera within a few days after arrival, 70 of whom died. The ship *Progress*, also from Liverpool, arrived two days later with 715 passengers, 44 of whom died from the disease. Any of these sites, Chicago, St. Louis or New York, may have been the source for the disease that appeared in Detroit that May.[2] The city authorities in Detroit, rightly concerned that the disease was making its way there, urged citizens to clean any "filth" from private premises, as well as to employ the liberal use of lime in helping "disinfect" the premises. Nevertheless, such precautions proved fruitless.

The first reported case of cholera in Detroit appeared on May 19, in a laborer living near May's Creek, one of the city waterways that closely paralleled the sewer along Savoyard. He was brought to St. Mary's Hospital suffering from fever, cramps and increasingly severe diarrhea. Despite medical treatment, he died three days later. A week later another case appeared, an Irishman living on Drummond Island in the Detroit River. After staying overnight at the railroad depot in the city, he developed the severe diarrhea typical of the disease, succumbing a week later. A third case, that of a pregnant woman, appeared at the same time. The woman appeared to be recovering when she developed puerperal fever, what we now understand is a streptococcal infection usually following childbirth; this infection proved fatal.[3]

Detroit's mayor, Oliver Hyde, seemed to exploit the developing epidemic as a means to enrich his own coffers, advocating the use of something called Tonic Liver Pills. Even the local newspaper was caught by surprise:

> A handbill that had been circulating through the city, purportedly to have been issued by the Mayor, and addressed to the citizens, announcing that the cholera was prevailing in the city, and advising the use of "Conger's Magic Regulator and Tonic Liver Pills" as a certain preventive and cure, we supposed the thing was a very ingenious trick of the proprietor of the medicine to obtain it for notoriety and sale. We did not for a moment imagine that the Mayor, either in his official or individual capacity, could be guilty of such folly and outrage as to issue the handbill, or connive at its issue.... And when, on Saturday evening, Mayor Hyde called upon us, and assured us that his signature to the handbill had been obtained under misapprehen-

9. Epidemic of 1854

sion, and that he designed to make no such publication, we gave him credit for candor and truth, though we saw no way to excuse his imprudence and folly.

Murder will out! We have evidence, entirely satisfactory to ourselves, that the issue of this handbill was a deliberate act of the Mayor, and that the said Mayor is a joint proprietor of "Conger's Magic Regulator and Tonic Liver Pills"!! Thus the milk in the coconut is accounted for. Thus the conduct of the Mayor is explained.

Was there ever a more flagrant breach of the public confidence, by a similar officer, under similar circumstances? The Mayor was not content with merely sending out a bald falsehood, intended to produce panic among our citizens, and calculated to injure the trade and commerce of the city by deterring people from coming in from the country, but he took a step which marks him as a wicked man at heart — as one who is willing to hazard, aye, endanger human life, for the base purpose of putting money in his own pocket.[4]

It was not only members of the press who were upset with the mayor. The practicing physicians of Detroit also met that June 17, producing a resolution in which "the undersigned physicians of this city, strongly express our disapprobation of the action of our Mayor, and regard it as an imposition upon the public, well calculated to produce the disease where it would not otherwise have existed."[5] The physicians denied, as well, even the existence of an outbreak beyond that of a few isolated cases.

So what was the result of the issuance of the handbill? William Conger, the co-proprietor and friend of the mayor, attempted to absolve Hyde of any wrongdoing. Hyde's response was that since he was already using the elixir, he assumed he was merely endorsing the product when Conger asked him to sign the handbill. In the end, the mayor remained in office, and the story was subsequently forgotten. But there was a larger, overriding issue in place. Despite the denials by the authorities, including the city physicians, cholera had appeared in the city and was spreading among the population even as the story was being debated. Ironically, one of the physicians who had signed the resolution disavowing Hyde's and Conger's elixir, a resolution that denied the presence of any significant outbreak of cholera, was Dr. Zina Pitcher. Pitcher had been treating patients, largely without success, who had been appearing with cholera for over a month by this time. Pitcher himself had called attention to the presence of disease:

Early in June the attention of the city government was called to this subject by the occurrence of a sudden death, reported as cholera, on Atwater Street near the Hydraulic Tower. From inquiries made of other practitioners, I learned that cholera had already acquired domicile in the 4th and 7th wards of the city, among the newly arrived immigrants, particularly from Holland, where it had held such a relation to Typhus or Ship-fever [likely typhus], that it was often difficult to determine in a given case, which of the morbid elements held the predominance. By the middle of this month [June] the epidemic influence of cholera was firmly established. From this time to the first of August there was no appreciable mitigation of its force.[6]

As had been the situation in previous epidemics, the authorities, including the major physicians of Detroit, preferred to underplay the presence of the disease. In part, of course, this was to prevent significant panic from developing, which might in turn result in the inhabitants of the city fleeing to other areas and carrying the disease with them.[7] The Common Council had acknowledged Pitcher's report—referring only to the account of a physician—but concluded "there is no ground whatever of alarm; and the authorities are performing but a simple duty in taking early precautionary measures."[8]

Concerns were raised about the safety of the city water. Pitcher defended the quality of the city water in a report placed with the water commissioners. Included was an analysis carried out by Professor Silas Douglass, a chemistry colleague of Pitcher's from the University of Michigan, and who had studied medicine under Pitcher at one time. Douglass found no significant levels of impurities in the water he tested, the source of which was a pipe extending some 25 feet into the Detroit River.[9] In the 1850s there would have been little thought or incentive to test for sewage contamination beyond any obvious visible particulates. Certainly there was no basis at the time to test for the presence of microbial contamination, tests that are routinely carried out in the present day in checking for any input of sewage (e.g., coliform counts). However, one might have used the nitrogen content as a surrogate marker for the presence of even small amounts of sewage, had Douglass been so inclined. There is no evidence he did so. Pitcher's conclusion regarding the water supply at this time, 1854, was that it was pure. Furthermore, though the Sanatary (sic) Police of the city was in "wretched condition" at the time of the outbreak of cholera, the city had "adopted a system of sewers sufficiently extensive to carry off the surface water of the districts through which they extend."[10]

9. Epidemic of 1854

Among the challenges faced by the city's physicians was distinguishing cholera from other, too often common, waterborne diseases, in particular typhoid fever and dysentery. The underlying reason behind the spread of cholera — sewage contamination of the water supply — also contributed to the outbreak of typhoid and dysentery, illnesses endemic to many cities in the nineteenth century. Typhus, which was not a waterborne disease but one spread by lice or ticks, compounded the difficulties in coming to a proper diagnosis, since the symptoms in some instances were similar to those of the aforementioned diseases. Pitcher attempted to distinguish the different illnesses among his patients:

> Among the arrivals from Europe, there was one man who reached this place late in the winter. As his case shows ... how the types of disease become blended during the prevalence of an epidemic meteoration, I will describe it briefly. On the voyage out, about seventy of his fellow passengers had died of a disease which, according to the newspapers, resembled both Cholera and Typhus Fever. It was attended by intense pain in the abdomen, violent cramps and coldness of the extremities, to which would succeed nausea and collapse, without diarrhea. During the summer, but in a milder form, I have met with many analogous cases. The man himself was unwell when he left quarantine in New York. On arriving here he was very ill and applied for admission to the Hospital. The pains in his case were relieved by discharges of blood resembling prune juice, and large in quantity.... Under the endermic use of capsicum [cayenne pepper, still used today for relief of some forms of nausea] and carbonate of potash and the internal use, of small doses, of quinine ... the man recovered.
>
> By the 20th of June we had cases of Typhoid Fever approximating Cholera, and cases of Cholera ... so closely simulated Typhus Fever, that a person ignorant of the history of both, could not guess what had been the antecedent of either. Here let me remark that I make a distinction, which to my mind is clear, between Typhus and Typhoid Fevers. My post-mortem examinations this month (June) were mostly confined to Cholera subjects. The exceptions were those who died of Typhoid Fever.[11]

From here Pitcher described the results of his post-mortem examinations. Clearly there was severe abdominal involvement. What is missing in his descriptions is either the severe diarrhea nearly always characteristic of cholera, or the significant rash usually associated with typhus. One could make the case that what Pitcher has been diagnosing as cholera might in some patients actually have been typhoid fever. The reduced number of deaths among the ill may also suggest typhoid rather than cholera, since the former has a mortality rate closer to 25 percent, significantly lower than that associated with cholera.

The committee appointed by the Board of Health, consisting of the mayor, several aldermen, and physicians, whose job was to oversee causes of death as well as total internments, tried reassuring the public in another manner:

> Nearly all the mortality from cholera in our city, thus far, and a very large proportion of that from other diseases, has been confined to our foreign population — either from amongst those who have very recently emigrated to this country, (many, indeed, having just arrived here) or who have resided here, at the most, but a few years. The committee has no hesitation in saying that fully five-sixth of the deaths from cholera have been among people of the class referred to. Of the causes of this unusual mortality among our foreign population, the committee deem it unnecessary to remark. They are, undoubtedly, apparent to all our citizens.[12]

It was not difficult finding obvious examples in that foreign population. As an example, the Gronasen family from Norway emigrated to Canada in 1854, temporarily stopping in Quebec. From there they moved to Detroit, unfortunately timing the trip to coincide with the ongoing cholera outbreak. The father, Einar Gronasen, and youngest son developed cholera, dying shortly thereafter. The surviving members of the family migrated to Wisconsin, where both the mother, Berit, and a daughter, died from the disease.[13] The obvious implication here is that cholera was largely a disease prevalent among the foreigners now residing in the city. Even if this were true, the writer overlooked the contagious nature of the disease. The poverty that underlay the outbreak was not confined to only this population within the city, and cholera did not long remained confined to only a segment of the population.

Among the victims of cholera in Detroit at this time were Rabbi Samuel Marcus and the Reverend Professor Charles Fox. Marcus was hired in 1850 to officiate at Temple Beth El, established in September 1850 as the first synagogue in Michigan. The congregation initially met at the home of Sarah and Isaac Cozens near the corner of Congress and St. Antoine streets, but later moved to the upper floor of the store at 220 Jefferson Avenue owned by Jacob Silberman and Adam Hirsch. Marcus died at his home on St. Antoine Street. Professor Fox, ordained in the Episcopal Church, was a professor in the agricultural department at the

University of Michigan in Ann Arbor. At the time of his death, he had been the editor of the *Farmer's Companion and Horticultural Gazette*. Fox's death was one of 11 that occurred in Ann Arbor; in contrast, only a single death was reported in nearby Port Huron, the site of Fort Gratiot, infamous as the source of the 1832 epidemic. Dr. Cyrus M. Stockwell attributed the relatively few cases of the disease in Port Huron during the 1854 epidemic to the "porosity of the soil which favored the absorption of dew and rain, and also permitted the washing away of the fungoid growths, or germs." It was also alleged the same conditions prevented development of the cholera miasma in the city as well.[14] Stockwell had twice been president of the state medical society and was a prominent physician in that locale; his explanation therefore carried some credibility.

The epidemic in Detroit peaked between the latter weeks of June and the middle of August, though deaths continued to be reported throughout the following months. Children and pregnant women seemed to be particularly affected by an extreme form of the disease, coined Cholera Infantum in children by Pitcher.[15] In some instances the illness due to cholera was exacerbated by other infections, including erysipelas and puerperal fever (each a streptococcal infection); needless to say, mortality was very high in these circumstances.

Estimates of the number of deaths due to cholera in this epidemic were more accurate than those in the previous 1849 outbreak, in part because the instructions given to the Board of Health included the request for an accurate count of the number of interments. The estimate for June was 210 interments, for July, 781 interments, and for August, 456 interments. The greatest number of deaths in a 24-hour period took place on June 23, when 41 persons died. Pitcher himself acknowledged that of this total number (1,447), approximately 1,000 of the deaths were the result of cholera.[16] Pitcher also conceded he had limited knowledge as to the cause of the disease, again relying on the usual environmental characteristics that seemed to accompany such outbreaks.

> The earlier cases of Cholera in the epidemic of 1854 seemed to be traceable to the influence of local causes, such as stagnant water, overflowing vaults, heaps of decaying animal and vegetable matter, and the use of surface water drawn from superficial wells in parts of the city to which our hydraulic system has not yet been extended; but as the season advanced special causation

seemed to be lost sight of. Whether this is in any degree to be ascribed to the action of the city authorities in the abatement of nuisances, or in that of the Water Commissioners in extending free hydrants to the destitute parts of the city, involves in its decision a question we have not now time to discuss, viz., the consideration of the doctrine of zymosis [i.e., fungal infection as the cause], or the theory of fermentation, as applied to the propagation of disease, either in the increase in the morbid elements, in the person of the subject, or in the atmosphere by which he may be surrounded.[17]

Treatment of cholera remained a matter of choice for the physician, many being variations of what has previously been discussed. Each physician as well provided his own testimonials, standing by the belief that if the treatment did not kill the patient, and the patient subsequently recovered, the treatment must have been successful. Pitcher was no exception; as he was among the most eminent physicians in the city during this period, his treatments carried more credibility than others. His first step was to administer an emetic consisting of sodium chloride (salt) in an infusion of *Piper nigrum* (black pepper). This was followed by between ten and 20 grains of "chloride of hydragyrum" (literally, liquid silver — actually mercury).[18] Pitcher was also among the advocates of the regimen practiced at St. Mary's Hospital, where many of the cholera patients were treated. In addition to the aforementioned emetics, patients received a mixture of Syrup Rhei Aromatic, a rhubarb extract that may produce constipation, liquid ammonium acetate and opiated camphor. Pitcher was also an advocate of "dry cupping" in the gastric region of the patient. The procedure differs from bleeding in that no incision is made, so no blood is drawn. A hot cup is placed over the area, and as it cools the vacuum that is created draws the tissue into the cup, hopefully providing relief from any pain. Whether the procedure produced any improvement in the patient was debatable, but at least it would do no harm.

The principle behind the treatments was to evacuate (vomit) the substance associated with the symptoms of cholera, or whatever illness the patient might have encountered. Given the multitude of diseases associated with the sanitary conditions of the time, the symptoms may have represented many types of waterborne illnesses. The person might recover, and Pitcher stood by the effectiveness of his treatment, but it may very well not have been cholera from which the patient was suffering.

9. Epidemic of 1854

In New York, physicians still relied on the calomel treatment for cholera, repeating as often as necessary for the patient to retain the substance. A variation also utilized was an additional solution of camphor mixed with chloroform, with 10 to 20 drops repeatedly administered to the patient. Calomel, or mercurous chloride, had long been a popular medical treatment because of its alleged sedative properties, assuming the patient was even able to retain it. Dr. Adrian Vanderveer of the Franklin Street Cholera Hospital, a center opened as a result of the 1854 cholera epidemic in that city, was among the most vociferous of its advocates. Disregarding any purgative properties of the calomel, Vanderveer would continue to administer increasing doses until the patient retained the drug:

> It has frequently occurred that patients, both in hospital and private practice, have been seized with violent vomiting, purging, and cramps, which had, from their own statement, been kept up every ten minutes for one, two, and three hours; and, after taking sixty grains of calomel, have not vomited or purged for six, ten, and twelve hours after; and, in two or three instances in the hospital, after waiting twelve hours, resorted to mild enema to open the bowels. I have found calomel in large doses more sedative (than cathartic) in its effects, and that its cathartic actions [i.e., diarrhea] does not increase in proportion to the increase in dose.[19]

Vanderveer pointed out that his treatment had saved nearly one-third of his patients with cholera. Of course with the mortality associated with untreated cholera being approximately 70 percent, it would appear Vanderveer's treatment had minimal effect. And as briefly addressed in a previous chapter, calomel, being a mercury compound, was itself inherently toxic.

Others produced their own variations on the calomel treatment. Dr. A.G. Lawton, an Illinois physician, had tried calomel along with camphor, opium and capsicum on his patients, but remained unsatisfied with the results. Calomel, Dover's powder, a combination of ipecac and opium, and quinine were also utilized. After administration of this combination Lawton added castor oil and spirits of turpentine. When, or if, the patient began to recover, Lawton found white sugar completed the medical process. Allegedly he had reasonably good results with this combination of medications.[20] It perhaps should be noted that Dr. Lawton was expelled the following year from the Illinois State Medical Society for selling patent medicines and other nostrums, and publishing "unprofessional matter" in newspapers.

An even more radical treatment was suggested at this time, utilizing acids. Dr. W.J. Anderson prescribed "mineral acids," specifically nitric acid and sulphuric acid. The reasoning was convoluted but seemed sufficient in the physician's mind to justify this form of treatment:

> That oxygen is given off most rapidly from the blood in cholera, may be observed, even during life, by the speedy oxidation of the tissues, giving rise to that horrible emaciation so characteristic of the complaint; again, the cold and blue-colored surface at a later period shows too plainly the large amount of oxygen which has been expended, and the fearful quantity of carbon which is now circulating in the slowly flowing blood. The patient has now a fluid passing through his blood vessels, somewhat similar to that which exists in cyanosis, insufficiently stimulating to the nervous system, and consequently blunting the mental faculties (though not by any means obliterating them).... Can a remedy then be found, which will readily yield up its oxygen and supply that element to the impure blood, and at the same time, by its astringent properties, tend to check the enormous exudation which takes place from the mucous surface of the intestinal canal? In our present state of knowledge, some of the mineral acids appear to be the best adapted to this purpose; and for certain reasons ... a combination of nitric with sulphuric acid seems to me to be preferable to any other.... The large amount of oxygen contained in the nitro-sulphuric acid will be called into play.... Oxygen is the important agent which must be called into play to produce a beneficial effect.... In a large number of casual cases of diarrhea, lately applying for relief, as well as many others which have occurred under my own treatment ... this remedy has proven speedily effective with some very few exceptions; the diarrhea and vomiting have ceased, and griping and cramps, when present, have been almost immediately removed.[21]

This opinion was seconded by one Dr. Fuller of St. George's Hospital in London, who prescribed a regimen of sulphuric and nitric acid mixed with camphor. Each testified that in no cases did the mixtures fail to relieve vomiting, cramps and diarrhea characteristic of cholera.[22] In both instances the physicians had mistaken the cyanotic color as being entirely the result of loss of oxygen, rather than the extreme depletion of fluid resulting from the extreme diarrhea.

The 1850s also found a growing interest among some physicians in the practice of homeopathy. Homeopathy, described briefly in an earlier chapter, is based upon the premise that drugs that produce symptoms resembling those of the disease being treated may actually be beneficial in curing that disease. The practice originated with a German physician, Samuel Hahnemann, as early as the 1790s. Hahnemann felt — correctly — that procedures such as bloodletting or the administration of toxic "medicines" were more likely to harm the patient than provide any benefit. There was some basis for his belief in the benefit of the "similar" in treating disease. While translating William Cullen's work *Materia Medica* into German, he found a reference to the use of cinchona bark, a component of which is quinine, as a treatment for malaria. Hahnemann tested this on himself, chewing a large quantity of the bark extract after which he developed chills, which he interpreted as symptoms analogous to those of malaria. The "symptoms" were likely an allergic response to the drug. Nevertheless Hahnemann applied the concept of *similia similibus curentur*—"let likes be cured by likes"— to the treatment of disease in general.[23] Since many of the immigrants arriving in New York, Detroit and elsewhere were German, homeopathy was a particularly popular medical alternative during these years. With the reality that standard medical treatments were as likely to produce unpleasant, even life-threatening, side effects, and usually provided no beneficial effect anyway, one must concede that homeopathy at least did no harm to the patient. The practice of homeopathy continues even in the present day.

To give Hahnemann his due he was not far from being correct in some of his assumptions as they pertained specifically to cholera. He was a proponent of the contagious nature of the disease, laying out his argument through the use of observation and common sense:

> Two opinions, exactly opposite to each other prevail on this subject [of contagion vs. miasmatic]. One party considers the pestilence as only epidemic, of atmospheric-telluric nature, just as though it were merely spread through the air, from which in that case there would be no protection. The other party denies this, and holds it to be communicable by contagion only, and propagated from one individual to another.... The first has the most obstinate defenders, who adduce the fact that when the cholera has broken out at one extremity of the town, it may the very next morning be raging at the other extremity, consequently the infection may only be present in the air; and that they (the physicians) are in their own persons proofs of the non-contagious character of the cholera, seeing that they generally remain unaffected by it and in good health, although they are daily in personal communication with those dying of cholera, and have even tasted the matter they ejected and the blood out of their veins, lain down in their beds, and so forth. This foolhardy, disgusting procedure they allege to be the *experimentum cruces*,

that is to say, an incontrovertible truth of the non-contagious nature of cholera, that it is not propagated by contact, but is present in the atmosphere, and for this reason attacks individuals in widely distant places.

A fearfully pernicious and totally false assertion! [Italics in original.] Were it the fact that this pestilential disease was uniformly distributed throughout the atmosphere, like the influenza which recently spread over all Europe, then the many cases reported by all the public journals would be quite inexplicable, where small towns and villages [Hahnemann is referring to the current outbreak in Europe] in the vicinity of the murderously prevalent cholera, which, by the unanimous efforts of all their inhabitants, kept themselves strictly isolated, like a besieged fortress, and which refused to admit a single person from without — inexplicable, I repeat, would be the perfect exemption of such places from the ravages of the cholera.... How could the exemption been possible had the cholera been distributed throughout the atmosphere?[24]

Hahnemann still had to explain the sudden appearance of cholera in isolated settings, such as passengers or sailors on board ships. Here he qualified his belief in a purely contagious origin for the disease, falling back on the presence of a miasma which acted in conjunction with the contagion. Even so, his explanation for this characteristic of an outbreak — its appearance in isolated settings, and even the seemingly lesser incidence among physicians—came very close to the modern understanding of the disease. Infected individuals—sailors—do not become carriers. However in some individuals an infection may produce only mild, or delayed, symptoms. Hahnemann also applied some understanding of immunity, that a mild attack may protect the individual against further infection:

The only fact brought forth by [Christoph Wilhelm] Hufeland against my proofs (viz., that on board an English ship in the open sea ... that had had no (?) communication with the town, two sailors were suddenly seized with the cholera) proves nothing, for it is not known how near the ship came to the infected town, so that the sphere of the miasm-exhalation from the town, although diluted, might yet have reached and infected the sailors, who were still unused to the miasm, especially if they, as is often the case, were rendered more susceptible to it from intemperance.... On board ships—in those confined spaces, filled with mouldy watery vapors, the cholera-miasm finds a favourable element for its multiplication, and grows into an enormously increased brood of those excessively minute, invisible, living creatures, so inimical to human life, of which the contagious matter of the cholera most probably consists—on board these ships, I say, this concentrated aggravated

9. Epidemic of 1854

miasm kills several of the crew; the others, however, being frequently exposed to the danger of infection, and thus gradually habituated to it, at length become fortified against it, and no longer liable to be infected. These individuals, apparently in good health, go ashore, and are received by the inhabitants without hesitation into their cottages, and ere they have time to give an account of those who have died of the pestilence on board the ship, those who have approached nearest to them are suddenly carried off by the cholera. The cause of this is undoubtedly the invisible cloud that hovers closely around the sailors who have remained free from the disease, and which is composed of probably millions of those miasmatic animated beings, which, at first developed on the broad marshy banks of the tepid Ganges [in India], always searching out in preference the human being to his destruction and attaching themselves closely to him, when transferred to distant and even colder regions become habituated to these also, without any diminution either of their unhappy fertility or of their fatal destructiveness.... Those who are not debilitated, and have kept at some distance from the stranger who is surrounded by the cholera miasm, suffered only a mild attack from the miasmatic exhalation hovering about in a more diluted form; their vital force could easily ward off the weaker attack and master it, and when they subsequently came nearer it their system had by this time become somewhat habituated to the miasm, retained the mastery over it, and even when these persons at length approached nearer or quite close to the infected stranger, their vital force had thus become so fortified against it, that they could hold intercourse with him with perfect impunity, having now become completely uninfectable by the contagious principle of the cholera.... When first called to a cholera patient, the physician, somewhat timid as yet, as is but reasonable, either tarries at first in the antechamber (in the weaker atmosphere of the miasmatic exhalation) or if he enters the patient's room prefers keeping at some distance, or standing at the door, orders the nurse in attendance to do this or the other to the patient, he then prudently soon takes his departure promising to return again shortly; in the meantime he usually goes about a little in the open air, or goes home and has some refreshment. His vital force, which at the first short visit at some distance from the patient, was only moderately assailed by the diluted miasm, recovers itself completely in the meantime ... so that at last the physician is completely hardened against even the most poisonous cholera miasm at the bedside, and rendered quite uninfectable by this pestilence.[25]

Of course Hahnemann was incorrect in his seemingly wide application of protection of the attending physician. Physicians often did become infected while treating patients; while it is unknown how frequently any medical personnel utilized (today's) standard sanitary procedures, one might easily understand that a physician who became soiled while examining a patient might at least wash his hands (sometimes) upon leaving the site. But the physician or nurse, Hahnemann noted in his description of cholera, could also serve as the vector of transmission of the disease:

> It is not, they [physicians and nurses] say, the least catching. This presumptuous, inconsiderate, and perfectly untrue assertion has already cost thousands their lives, who in their ignorance, and quite unprepared, either approached the cholera patient suddenly, or came in contact with these cholera physicians (who do not treat with camphor) or their nurses. For such physicians and nurses, fortified in this manner against the miasm, now take away with them in their clothes, in their skin, in their hair, probably also in their breath, the invisible (probably animated) and perpetually reproductive contagious matter surrounding the cholera patient they have just visited, and this contagious matter they subconsciously and unsuspectingly carry along with them throughout the town and to their acquaintances, whom it unexpectedly and infallibly infects, without the slightest suspicion on their part of the source. Thus the cholera physicians and nurses are the most certain and frequent propagators and communicators of contagion far and wide.[26]

Hahnemann was willing to apply his contagion-miasm theory to the treatment of cholera as well. His recommendation was that physicians apply liberally camphorated spirits (camphor) both on themselves for protection and on the patient as well in order to cure the disease. At the same time, Hahnemann excoriated those physicians who continue the traditions of treating cholera with bloodletting or (as he recognized even in the nineteenth century) toxic chemicals.

> If the physicians would but take warning, and, rendered uninfectable by taking a few drops of the camphorated spirit, approach (ever so quickly) the cholera patient, in order to treat him at the commencement of his sickening with this medicine ... which alone is efficacious, and which most certainly destroys the miasm about the patient.... But these physicians despise this; they prefer going on killing their patients in crowds by pouring into them large quantities of aqua-fortis [nitric acid solution] and opium, by bloodletting, and so forth, or giving the camphor mixed with so many obstructing and injurious matters, that it can scarcely do any good, solely to avoid giving the simple, pure (efficacious) solution of camphor.... They seem to prefer delivering over all mankind to the gravedigger, to listening to the good counsel of the new purified healing art.[27]

In December 1854 the Detroit Medical Society established a committee, the function of which was to produce a report summarizing the diseases prevalent in Detroit and surrounding areas that year. The report was then to be presented to the State Medical Society. The report was to list and describe any epidemics that had taken place during the previous three years (1851–1854), when they began and subsequently ended, and in which portions of the region they had broken out. Given constraints on time — the report was to have been completed by the following month — the committee chose to focus primarily on the present year, 1854.[28]

Not surprisingly, the primary illnesses during the winter months were either waterborne illnesses such as typhoid fever or the types of contagious illnesses prevalent even in modern times: "croup" (primarily colds or influenza), streptococcal infections, including rheumatic fever, and pneumonia. During the early spring, diarrheal diseases such as dysentery became more common. The diseases prevalent in the city changed in May with the first appearance of cholera, as reported by Dr. Edward Batewell (Batwell) on the 18th. Other victims were observed by Dr. Zina Pitcher, as described earlier. During the time cholera was present in the city, between May and the end of October, over 1,000 persons had succumbed to the disease. Other illnesses reported during this period included smallpox, brought by "German emigrants," rheumatism, and the "most commonly reported diseases" such as phthisis (tuberculosis), neuralgia, menorrhagia and pleurisy.

The 1,000 deaths attributed to cholera represented a significant increase from the newborn observed during the 1834 outbreak. Given the population of the city at that time, some 35,000 persons, approximately 3 percent of the population died, significantly less than the 7–10 percent that had died during the previous outbreak. The media later had its own view of the origin and extent of the outbreak: "As usual the first cases occurred in low and filthy places, but it gradually spread, and for the month of June the number of deaths did not exceed two or three per day. During July the deaths from cholera averaged 12 per day. On several days the deaths ranged from 35 to 40. After August 1 the mortality was evidently on the decrease, the average deaths per day being from two to three until September 12 when the last deaths occurred."[29]

10

Epidemic of 1866: New York, Detroit and Beyond

The understanding of disease by medical practitioners sat on a cusp in the immediate aftermath of the Civil War. The germ theory of disease, the scientific concept that infectious disease is the result of infection by microscopic organisms, still remained a decade or more in the future. Nevertheless, observations in the biological sciences were taking place that would ultimately provide the background to that theory. French chemist Louis Pasteur was even then demonstrating the role of infectious agents in silkworm disease, as well as the role played by microscopic organisms in the fermentation reactions that contributed to the spoilage of food. Further, in refuting theories of spontaneous generation, the belief that life could form spontaneously in the presence of specific food items, i.e., life developing from nonlife, Pasteur demonstrated that microorganisms existed in the air itself. The conflict between "miasmatists," those who believed disease developed from odors or characteristics of the atmosphere, and "contagionists," the belief that disease was contagious and spread directly from person to person, would continue for several decades. But by the mid to late 1860s an increasing proportion of physicians were developing a better understanding of the nature of illness. The use of quarantine in attempts to isolate victims of diseases such as cholera or smallpox was a direct example of the growing belief in some form of infectious substance. Even in the absence of definitive evidence for an infectious agent that we would recognize today, other applications of cleanliness were being introduced and practiced. In Vienna, Ignaz Semmelweis, a physician at Vienna General Hospital, had proposed some years earlier that puerperal fever among women was the result of physicians carrying the disease agent with them when examining patients; Semmelweis was able to significantly decrease the incidence of the disease by requiring

10. Epidemic of 1866

that physicians wash their hands between patients. Similar conclusions were presented by New England physician Oliver Wendell Holmes, Sr., after his own observation that hospital physicians were transmitting the disease directly from patient to patient. The accusation was certainly highly controversial, the idea that physicians themselves were causing puerperal fever and condemning these women to a miserable death. Semmelweis and Holmes were later proven correct, but only subsequent to the infectious agents, members of the bacterial category of streptococci, being isolated and observed. Cholera too would later be shown by Robert Koch to be the result of infection, not the result of a miasma emanating from the earth. But in the year of 1866 Koch had just been graduated from medical school, and such discoveries lay in the future.

Medical care in the city of Detroit continued to evolve as well, commensurate with an increase in population, which now surpassed 50,000 persons in 1860, and would approach 70,000 by the end of the decade. Several years after the demise of the Wayne County Medical Society in 1851, another short-lived attempt was made to revive the organization. However, in March 1858 the society was once again dissolved, not due to the issue of medical licensing that had been the point of contention earlier, but over the question of whether a member could advertise his services to the general public. The miscreant apparently felt that since members of other professions such as those in the practice of law were perfectly free to do so, he had every right to advertise as well. The arguments devolved into recriminations in which members accused each other of lying or of undercutting their prices to eliminate competition, and even playing to friends among the media who would provide testimonials and bragging rights for the most mundane cases: "Dr. So-and-So attended with his usual grace and dignity, and performed the operation in a highly artistic and professional style."[1]

The onslaught of the war in 1861 resulted in an extreme shortage of physicians, not only in Detroit but in civilian centers throughout the country. A significant proportion of physicians and surgeons enlisted in the army. Some of the city of Detroit's most prominent older physicians remained in practice during these years, or were assigned duties there. Zina Pitcher and David Farrand were attendant physicians at St. Mary's Hospital in Detroit, founded in 1845 and at the time of the war the sole public hospital in the state. Following his graduation from the College of Physicians and Surgeons in New York City, Farrand had enlisted in the army as a surgeon, and was subsequently posted in Detroit. There he was assigned to St. Mary's Hospital, which in 1863 was designated as a military hospital since the majority of the patients at the hospital were wounded soldiers during these years.

The land for another military hospital on Woodward Avenue, west of downtown, was donated in 1863 by Walter Harper and Nancy Martin. What became known as Harper Hospital was constructed in 1864 as a wooden building flanked by several cottages; the hospital trustees were required to treat invalid soldiers at no expense to the patient even following the war, creating what in effect were the first such veteran's hospitals. Farrand was commissioned as assistant surgeon in the army, and served as medical director at Harper until after the war. After resigning from the army he joined Pitcher in private practice. Farrand subsequently served as president of the board of health for the city.

In 1866 attempts were once again carried out to revive both the state medical society as well as the Wayne County Medical Society. On May 15 a meeting was called by Pitcher and several other city physicians to arrange for delegates to meet the first week of June in Detroit for the purpose of organizing a new state medical society. Approximately 100 prospective members met on June 5. Dr. Moses Gunn was elected interim president, and among the committees established was one on admission to membership, the function of which was to ensure that any future members were indeed practicing physicians. Once the organization convened, Dr. Cyrus Stockwell from Port Huron was elected the first permanent president of the new society, which continues today as the Michigan State Medical Society.

On May 30 seventeen Detroit physicians and one physician from Northville met in the mayor's office for the purpose of re-establishing the county medical society as well. Zina Pitcher was elected president, and a fee of $3 was agreed upon for physicians wishing to become members. The function of the society centered on the discussion of general medical topics and the importance of maintaining a system of ethics among the membership. The goal was to include participation of physicians throughout the county, not just the city of Detroit. While physicians in the surrounding communities expressed initial support for the society, difficulties in transportation and waning interest in the future did not bode well for its success any more than in the past. This time the Wayne County Medical Society would survive for a decade.

Though cholera continued to devastate much of the world in the period between 1854 and 1865, other than a few isolated cases Detroit was spared another epidemic. In part this was the recognition that improved sanitation, even beyond any improvement it provided in the quality of life, could mitigate the extent of an outbreak. This was proven convincingly during the 1854 outbreak in New York City, during which that city's board of health, reconstituted as a result of the presence of cholera, enforced sanitation procedures. Fewer than 600 persons died in the city during that epidemic, a considerable number but a proportion far fewer than experienced in previous outbreaks.

Concern that with the spread of cholera elsewhere in the world, including eastern Canada, a new epidemic might again appear in Detroit, the Board of Health met on September 7, 1865, at city hall to discuss sanitation issues in the city. Dr. William Brodie, the president of the board, opened the proceedings by laying out before the members the situation. As described in the media:

> Alleys in the upper part of the city were comparatively clean, but those in the lower part, particularly where business was transacted, abounded in filth. In the first and second wards, fronting on Woodbridge Street, this was particularly noticeable. Among the whole which he had visited there were only two clean. The alley between Cass and First Streets, first north of Jefferson Avenue, was an intolerable nuisance, and others which he could name were in an extremely filthy state. He said that the history of the cholera was this time different from all the others. It appeared to be confined to the Mediterranean basin, but was possible traveling westward. [He was correct.] There had occurred some cases of cholera in the city in the summer which were as bad as any in 1854, and attended with all the symptoms of the virulent disease. The city should be thoroughly cleansed, because when the epidemic was upon us it was no time to take precautionary measures.[2]
>
> "From the incomplete state of our system of lateral sewage, and the extensive neglect of the proper and decent drainage of private premises ... it is indispensable ... that all parties be notified as soon as may be by the proper authority, to drain their premises thoroughly into the nearest sewer which may be reasonably accessible, and that all such drains shall be fitted with a stench trap.

Other resolutions requested that health inspectors for the wards monitor the cleanup of unsanitary conditions and observe for the presence of any disease, and that the board of police commissioners "detail at least one additional member of the police force to examine and make report of all nuisances throughout the city."[3]

In an attempt to address the concerns raised at the September meeting, Brodie called for a special meeting which was held at city hall on November 10. The president again raised his concerns that another outbreak of cholera in Detroit would likely take place in the near future, and that immediate measures must be taken "to counteract its pernicious influence" even though it was not yet the season for the disease to appear; among his concerns was the presence of cholera on a ship, the *Atalanta*, that had recently docked in New York harbor. Brodie recommended that a subcommittee should be appointed by the board to provide recommendations for preventing the appearance or spread of the disease. He also followed up the recommendation from the previous meeting that both a health official and member of the police should examine sanitary conditions in the wards and prosecute anyone failing to address those conditions. Finally, Brodie recommended that a city dispensary should be established to provide needed supplies in the event of an outbreak. Zina Pitcher offered a resolution that a committee of five should be appointed to oversee measures that would "promote the public health and prevent the introduction and spread of that appalling disease." The resolution was adopted, with Pitcher appointed to the committee.[4]

The decisions made by the board of health had the support of the local media, particularly in light of the presence of the disease in New York.

> Under these circumstances, it was eminently right and proper that the Board of Health should meet and consult as to any and what means should be taken to mitigate, if not to avoid the danger.... As we have heretofore suggested, cleanliness is most efficacious. But few of our citizens realize how much dirt and filth is accumulated in the lanes and alleys under the basements of their houses.... A thorough inspection only can reveal it, and this should be the course adopted by the Board, and it is one which commends itself to all. It is, we are aware, often inconvenient to submit one's premises to a thorough inspection, and particularly the drainage. In order to get at it the necessity often exists to take up floors, and these cannot always be replaced with the same material, as it is frequently so far rotted and used up as to be worthless. But it is far better to submit to the inconvenience and loss than to find too late that the necessary precautions have not been taken."[5]

10. Epidemic of 1866

A special meeting of the board was held on November 23 to hear the recommendations as presented by Pitcher on behalf of the committee. The meeting began with a summary of sanitary conditions in the city. While portions of the city were satisfactory, other streets were characterized by filthy ditches that needed to be drained, stagnant water, compost, privies not connected with the public sewer and even the filth originating with the Michigan Central Railroad cattle-yards. Other unsanitary material consisted of the slops and swill thrown out for pigs and geese.

Pitcher reminded the board that a means to deal with the problem in the face of the approaching cholera was already in place: water commissioners with the authority to connect homes to the sewer system, police commissioners with authority to enforce the decrees of the Common Council, and the Board of Health as well. Pitcher, on behalf of the committee, made several specific recommendations: first, the appointment of a health physician "to cooperate with the sanitary inspectors to thoroughly explore the whole city"; second, that "occupants of all premises contiguous to the sewers be required to drain them by making connections"; third, that the city should "cause all hydrants which allow water to escape upon the surface of the ground to be repaired"; fourth, "that the ordinance in relation to privies be rigorously enforced, by requiring them to be drained into the sewers or thoroughly cleansed; and fifth, where occupants or owners of premises are known to be unable to incur the expense of draining or cleansing them we would aid them by an appropriation of the public funds or by making an appeal to private munificence for their relief." In order to implement the resolutions, the board recommended that the Common Council print copies of the recommendations on circulars to be placed throughout the city as well as in the media to inform the public of the board's concern, and to request their aid in addressing the unsanitary conditions which had to be eliminated[6]:

Cholera

We trust that the authorities and citizens of Detroit will do their utmost to thoroughly cleanse every portion of the city. Every citizen has a direct interest in this matter. The cholera permits no one to repeat Cain's question: "Am I my brother's keeper?" with impunity. Personal cleanliness is not enough; the air laden with the impure vapors which reek from filthy alleys and stagnant pools in the remotest parts of the city may bring the pestilence to inhabitations in which the utmost cleanliness prevails. An appeal to the people of Detroit to see that every portion of the city is thoroughly cleansed is an appeal not merely to the philanthropy, but the desire of personal safety to every citizen.[7]

The city was only partially successful in addressing the sanitation problem. Pockets of "filth" remained. But the greater problem was the question of dealing with the enormous amount of sewage that was ever-present in a nineteenth century city. By the latter years of the decade Pasteur's work demonstrating the presence of life, "germs," in the atmosphere was generally known in the medical field. While the link between these microscopic agents and disease had not yet been established, their mere presence in the air was still considered a concern. Even though many of the privies in the city had been connected to the greater disposal system by the time of the outbreak in 1866, most of the sewage was still passed into the Detroit River, where it contaminated much of the water used by the population of the city.

The challenge of sewage disposal was pointed out by Dr. Samuel Duffield, the professor of chemistry at Detroit Medical College; his work was discussed in the previous chapter. Duffield estimated approximately ten tons of solid human fecal material passed into the city sewers on a daily basis, as well as 440,000 pounds of urine. This did not include fecal waste from animals, or runoff from the slaughter houses:

> At almost every corner these wide-gaping mouths are pouring forth a vapor, unseen, insidious, more to be dreaded than the fumes of the Stygian Lake.... As there are rarely stench traps from the privies to the main sewers, the air passes up from the sewers at night (the external air being colder than the air in the sewer), and we have in this city the familiar odor of the sewers and privies from ten or eleven at night to eight-o-clock in the morning. It is a matter of fact that there are sources of the malignant cholera and cholera morbus, which attack our cities during the hot months; and if our city fathers would only consider it is absolutely necessary to bottle up the vapors of these sewer mouths, then we should have less sickness. An analysis of the air at this period shows it loaded with these poisonous germs, which we breathe in at night, to develop into dysentery, cholera morbus, and sometimes cholera.[8]

Duffield was mistaken in implying the presence of odors, miasmas, in the air as the direct cause of cholera. He was correct, however, in

10. Epidemic of 1866

implicating the ever-present sewage as the source of the outbreaks. That he did not at least suggest an infectious agent might be the source of the cholera is perhaps surprising, given that he was certainly aware such "zoo germs" were agents in other diseases: "The 'zoo germs' are carried into the blood through the lungs and developed in the system, producing the ague, remittent, and other fevers. Pasteur has shown conclusively the existence of this germ life. Crookes and others have proven the active poison of cattle disease was purely germinal, and have caught and examined under the microscope the various forms in the various stages of that loathsome evil."[9] Where Duffield failed to apply this information was in assuming the agent is inhaled, not swallowed, as is the case in cholera.

Duffield was far from the only educated scientist who failed to suspect the presence of an agent in food or water as the cause of cholera. Circumstantial evidence for the presence of an agent in water had been building for nearly two decades. In 1849 and again in 1854, British physician John Snow had linked the cholera outbreaks in London to contaminated water supplies. While he never demonstrated the presence of a specific organism in the water, he did suggest the presence of a "poison" in the excreta and stools of the patient, and suggested it was capable of reproducing itself in those who were subsequently infected. Most physicians were convinced that a cholera "poison" of some sort was to be found in the diarrhea. But here they diverged into those who felt the agent was sufficient in itself to propagate the disease, and those who believed that some form of "fermentation" was necessary. Something, perhaps a miasma of undefined form, had to be present in the air as well — the odor or smell of decomposing organic matter, including feces. Perhaps "a contaminated atmosphere — as in a tenement — must weaken the 'system' generally and thus predispose it to cholera."[10]

Since the incidence of cholera was commonly high in the German states during these pandemics, and the German educational system, particularly in field of medicine, was among the highest quality in the Western world, it is perhaps not surprising that many of the most advanced ideas about cholera would be found there. Max von Pettenkofer, German professor of hygiene and among the most prominent proponents on the importance of sanitation and hygiene in prevention of cholera, was one of the first to recognize the importance of fecal contamination in the development of the disease; where he was mistaken was in the failure to acknowledge the specific etiological role played by a biological agent, even after such an agent had been isolated by his colleague Robert Koch (see chapter 11). Pettenkofer believed that the diarrhea from a cholera victim did indeed play a role in spread of the disease, but that other putrescent factors in the soil were necessary as well; by this reasoning, cholera was not contagious. It should be kept in mind that in 1866 few diseases, and none in humans, were associated with microorganisms; otherwise it is difficult to understand how the medical minds of the time missed the role played by such organisms in disease. Cholera makes a perfect example. Professor Felix von Niemeyer, a professor of internal medicine at the University of Tubingen and a colleague of Von Pettenkofer, came as close as anyone to understanding the contagious nature of the disease. But here again his opinion was subject to the wisdom of the period:

> It is, on the one hand, certain that cholera is not communicated directly from one person to another even under circumstances of the greatest intimacy, but on the other hand, it is as certainly spread only by patients afflicted with the disease. The disease is propagated by the evacuations of individuals infected with cholera, probably in all, and certainly in most cases.... By means of one infected person in whom the disease has manifested itself only by a seemingly insignificant diarrhea, cholera can be conveyed to a hitherto healthy locality. This person may travel on and recover without further development of the disorder, but he has left behind him in the water-closet matter which may give rise to a most deadly epidemic. It is thus no longer inexplicable how the cholera in its wanderings takes no defined course, but spreads indifferently from west to east, from east to west, now with the wind and now against it, how it always follows the routes of travel, how it does not go from place to place in a shorter time than is required for men to travel the same distance, and how, since the building of railways it has been able to spread more quickly than before.[11]

Von Niemeyer showed a clear understanding of the role played by human "discharges" in the spread of cholera, which explained as well the path of the disease as it followed human travels. The railroads were the most modern contemporary method of conveyance, and as is true for airplane travel in our own times, also provided a mechanism for the wider and more rapid dissemination of disease. Von Niemeyer recognized that cholera rarely passed directly from person to person, as was the case for diseases like smallpox, mistaking the contagious nature of the disease in being unaware of the requirement that the cholera agent must be swallowed, not inhaled.

In the fall 1865 cholera was spreading through Europe, and using the previous outbreaks as precedent, most physicians felt it was merely a matter of time before it again reached the United States. Despite the war, the 1860s were still characterized by a continuation of the significant level of immigration to the United States that had begun as a consequence of the Irish famine 20 years earlier. By 1866, 20 percent of the population was foreign-born; one-third of these immigrants arrived from the German states, regions in which cholera was present.

The first, albeit brief, appearance of the disease on American shores occurred in November 1865. The ship *Atalanta* arrived in New York carrying passengers stricken with the disease. Attempts were made to reassure the public:

> The pestilence has not come to us on any first-class passenger ship, although such are constantly plying between our ports and the region in which the cholera rages. Another fact is that the cholera ... has only touched one class of passengers—those in the steerage ... a place in which the largest number of passengers that ever cross the seas are crowded like cattle on the way to market. It is even an exceptionally bad passage; for the ship does not come straight from her starting place to this port in the ordinary time. Her machinery got out of order. She stopped at a French port to have it repaired. And she has been out altogether thirty-four days. Add the discomforts, then, of an unusually long voyage to the ordinarily bad conditions of a steerage passenger, and we find an abundant explanation for unusual mortality—Bad or insufficient water and food, an overlong stay in the fetid atmosphere of the steerage, and the fright of the ignorant passengers of touching at a French port—all these are what constitute the "cholera" on the *Atalanta*.... Twenty deaths are the most reported by the worst story, and this is out of five hundred and four passengers, on a voyage of twenty-four days—less than a death a day. Does anyone believe that cholera would act that way? The cholera story will have one good effect if it makes us clean up our crowded and dirty places—the "steerage" of our cities—the only places where cholera has ever done any harm. It is to be hoped that it will not stimulate timid physicians into reporting as cholera every case of doubtful intestinal disease.[12]

Dr. Theo. McGraw, the translator of Niemeyer's article, applied that author's understanding in explaining the cholera outbreak on the *Atalanta*: "The course of the pestilence in its recent outbreak on the Atalanta can well be explained by Pettenkofer's theory. The disease sprung up in the steerage into which it may have been brought by one infected individual. The water-closets used by the different classes of passengers and crew on board ship are, as is well known, entirely distinct. While the cholera raged among the steerage passengers, not one person belonging to the crew or first cabin passengers was attacked."[13]

The British steamer *Atalanta* was the first of several ships that arrived in New York carrying passengers infected with cholera. It had departed London on October 10, arriving at Havre the following day. This is the port at which most of the steerage passengers joined the ship. Two German families on the ship had been staying at hotels, first in Paris at the hotel City of New York, and then at Havre at the hotels Weissen Lomni and Stuttgarder Hof. Several guests at each of these hotels had been hospitalized with what likely was cholera. On October 13 the *Atalanta* set sail for New York. On the first day after the ship left the port of Havre a child became ill with what was diagnosed as cholera, and died the following day. During the ensuing week, five additional members from the two families that had stayed at the hotels in Havre became ill and died from cholera. Other passengers soon developed cholera as well. By the time the ship reach New York on November 2, 60 cases of cholera were diagnosed; 15 died. Once the ship was in quarantine another eight passengers died, a total slightly higher than the estimate in the newspaper. There was no question that the disease was cholera.[14] The hospital ships *Falcon* and *Florence Nightingale* were assigned to provide medical aid for any passengers who became ill. Meanwhile, the *Atalanta* was ordered to the lower bay some miles from the city to wait out the quarantine. The *Atalanta* was thoroughly fumigated, and in mid-November, ten days after the last case of cholera appeared on the ship, the passengers were allowed to go on their way.

On November 26 seven deaths were reported on the ship *Hermani*. Like some of the victims on the *Atalanta*, the first victim had stayed at the Stuttgarder Hof in Havre. On December 12 the ship *Mary Ann* arrived, its voyage having originated at Havre; five deaths from cholera had occurred on the voyage to New York. Passengers thought to have been exposed to the disease were quarantined or hospitalized on Ward's Island, located in the East River. Sporadic cases appeared through mid-December, with the last recorded case diagnosed on December 20. According to the final reports from the Metropolitan Board of Health, any further outbreak was avoided due to the combination of the cold weather and the sanitary conditions that had been instituted.[15]

Cholera Arrives on the Mainland

The epidemic of 1866 in North America began in April with the presence of two passenger ships carrying victims of the disease. The first of these, the steamship *England*, arrived at the harbor in Halifax, Nova Scotia, on April 9. The ship had sailed from Liverpool on March 28 carrying 1,185 German and Irish emigrants, an additional 17 saloon-passengers, and a crew of 122 officers and men. Cholera appeared on April 1 with the death of a young boy. By the time the ship arrived at Halifax, one 160 cases of cholera had developed, with 46 deaths—some sources indicate 50 deaths—already having occurred. The death toll eventually rose to 267, most occurring among the passengers hospitalized at Halifax; as many as 25 persons died in one day.[16] Among the dead at Halifax was Dr. John Slayter, the city health officer who had been on board the *England*, and who succumbed to the disease on the 17th. Two additional physicians who had been with Slayter on the ship became ill but survived. Four members of a family in Halifax who had obtained clothing material from the ship also died from the disease, the only cases among persons not in direct physical contact with the passengers. The quarantine of the shop off McNabs Island near Halifax and the hospitalization of the *England*'s passengers prevented any further outbreak.[17]

During that same month of April, the first ship carrying passengers ill with cholera to dock at an American port, the steamship *Virginia*, entered New York harbor. The ship had departed from Liverpool on April 4 with 1,029 steerage passengers and 14 cabin passengers on board. After stopping briefly at Queenstown, Ireland, the ship arrived in New York on the 18th. At the time the *Virginia* had left Liverpool, several cases of mild diarrhea had been reported and largely ignored. Within a week after departure, however, several passengers developed the more severe diarrhea typical of cholera; by the following day the ship's surgeon acknowledged their illness as cholera. Over the course of the voyage, 36 steerage passengers and two members of the crew died from the cholera and were buried at sea; 46 additional passengers were ill when the ship arrived in New York. During the months of April and May the eventual total of cholera deaths, beginning with those aboard the *England* and *Virginia* and including the later arrivals of the ships *Union* and *Peruvian*, rose to 564.[18]

Passengers from the ships were to have been detained in quarantine for 22 days after the last case aboard their respective ships. However, with some 3,800 passengers in total from the four ships requiring detention, it is unlikely the quarantine was complete. Consequently any passengers who evaded quarantine, or who might have reached Manhattan during the quarantine period, could very well have included carriers. Regardless of how the victims became infected, the first illnesses or deaths from cholera in the city occurred on May 2 — nine persons living in tenements spread across the city — and all in places passengers from the ship might have frequented. In the words of Dr. John Swinburne, the health officer of the port, "The question may then be asked, if not traceable to quarantine, from what source did the infection in New York emanate? The answer is simple.... Others, among whom there had been no appearance of cholera during the voyage, but who came from European ports, where the disease is known to have prevailed, were mingling with their friends in New York in the course of from ten to fourteen days from the date of their probable exposure to cholera."[19] Passengers who had not been quarantined carried the disease with them, and either through socializing with friends or family — one in four New Yorkers by 1866 had been born in Ireland — or providing clothing, spread the disease into the city.

That the epidemic was not worse than it subsequently became was due to sanitation procedures instituted prior to the outbreak. Two years earlier, in 1864, pressure from physicians in the city resulted in wealthier citizens forming the Council of Hygiene and Public Health with the purpose of surveying the sanitary conditions prevalent in the city. The report produced by the council emphasized the extensive level of unsanitary conditions existing within the city and predicted that unless these conditions were addressed it would only be a matter of time before additional outbreaks of disease would occur. In 1865, for example, over 501,000 persons were crowded into 15,300 tenements. One such building was five stories high with the privies situated about five feet from the site and not connected to any sewer.[20]

10. Epidemic of 1866

In response both to the report and to the ongoing epidemic of cholera throughout Europe, the city government in February 1866 authorized the formation of the Metropolitan Board of Health, the job of which was to see to the clean-up of the city. Over the course of two months, 7,000 citations were issued to remove dead animal carcasses and manure, and to clean yards and streets.

Even as cholera appeared on the periphery of the city, the authorities attempted to reassure the public that matters were under control.

> The occurrence of what is probably cholera on a ship arriving in this port, and now in the Lower Bay [likely the *Virginia*], ought to occasion no anxiety or alarm in our community.... In all probability, it will be confined in Quarantine, as was the sickness of the *Atalanta*, and not appear in our city at all. We may reasonably hope that we have till the end of May or beginning of June to arrange the best quarantine — that is, to clean the city and remove its nuisances. The cholera, it must be remembered, is shorn of much of its terrors by modern science. Physicians tell us that not one case in a thousand is attacked by the disease without its premonitory symptom — the painless diarrhea — and this is a disturbance of the system readily managed.... The cholera is especially the punishment of neglect of sanitary laws; it is the curse of the dirty, the intemperate and the degraded. If it come to New York, we shall hear of it very little in the upper and well cared for portions of the city, the abodes of the middle and wealthy classes. It will revel in the cellars of the poor and among the packed tenement houses, and in those villages of shanties where pigs and human beings live huddled together. The slaughter houses and bone boiling establishments will be the nuclei of its ravages....
>
> The movement of the Board reported yesterday for securing the temporary barracks on the Battery [lower tip of Manhattan] is a wise one. It may be that whole blocks may have to be emptied of their tenants, and the people placed in tents (as was done with success in England) till the buildings are cleaned.[21]

While the media was praising the work of the board, at the same time it addressed the root causes of cholera — the conditions of the immigrant ships as well as the responsibilities of the authorities themselves:

> Human beings ought not to be packed together as they are now on these Liverpool and Irish steamers. Every steamer will become a nest of cholera if this practice continues. Why cannot an act of Congress regulate the cubic space for each passenger on scientific principles, now well known?
>
> But, vigorous as has been the Board of Health, there is one gigantic evil and stimulus to cholera which they have not as yet touched; we allude to the overcrowding of tenement houses and the cellar population. They ought to

pass the proposed resolutions requiring that every cellar with specified depth below the surface, and certain want of window space, used as a tenement, should be vacated after such and such a date. Then, at the time specified, the Police should proceed and turn the miserable wretches who inhabit them out into the street. Many of them would be better off in the Almshouse, or in tents, or in lodgings up-town, or in the suburbs.[22]

The situation on the emigrant ships was only marginally better in the 1860s than a decade earlier. During the early years of the century, much of the shipping between England and Canada was a by-product of the timber industry; Canadian wood was brought east across the ocean, while on the westward voyage the ships were largely empty. Never ones to miss out on a few extra sources of income, the owners constructed temporary passenger berths in the cargo holds by placing boards across the beams, thereby creating addition levels for increased numbers of passengers; the fees collected from the passengers often exceeded those obtained from the shipping of timber. On an average sized vessel, 250 to 300 passengers could be traveling on a deck "96 feet long, 26 feet across, and six feet high. The uncaulked deck floor — uncaulked because the decks were torn up to provide storage space for timber on the return voyage — became a collection point for filth and a snare for clothing, and the windowless hold a receptacle for cooking and body odors. Within a ten foot space on an unventilated deck, one passenger might be cooking food, another performing the offices of nature."[23] The wonder is not that cholera or other intestinal diseases occurred at all, but that they were not universal among this class of passenger.

When cholera did break out in May, the board oversaw the disinfection of those areas, almost exclusively among the poor, and the removal to hospitals of anyone having contact with the disease. Ultimately over 1,100 New Yorkers died from cholera between May and November. But the actions of the board prevented the outbreak, at least that portion confined to the city, from becoming even worse.[24]

Cholera: New York to Detroit

Between the beginning of May and the middle of July, 21 deaths were reported in New York as the result of the cholera outbreak. All were in the regions of the city visited or associated with the recent emigrants.

10. Epidemic of 1866

On July 3, a death was recorded among the army troops in Fort Columbus on Governor's Island near the tip of Manhattan, and the site of an army post that remained until 1966. Most of the men stationed there were recent recruits, and from there the inductees would be sent throughout the United States, a result of reorganization within the army following the end of the war. Soon after the first victim, a man from Minneapolis, Minnesota, with no known exposure, was admitted to the hospital, a second recruit was diagnosed with the disease. Several of the men were transferred to Hart's Island northeast of Manhattan in Long Island Sound, but here again the disease broke out. Within a few weeks over 180 cases were diagnosed among the soldiers, with 78 deaths.[25]

On July 14, the steamship *San Salvador* docked at Governor's Island, where 476 troops boarded for transport south. At the time the ship reached Tybee Island off the coast of Savannah, Georgia, 25 cases of cholera were reported, with three deaths. By the beginning of August more than 200 cases of cholera had developed, with 116 deaths; nine persons living on the island also became ill with cholera. The presence of the outbreak produced panic among the troops, resulting in a significant number of desertions during this period, many of whom hid throughout the island, or even ran as far as Savannah itself, some ten miles away. From a soldier's letter:

> We landed 470 troops on Tybee Island, and yesterday [July 23] eighty of the members answered to their names. They were so completely demoralized that 100 deserted and are scattered all over these islands, and they say that some have even got to Savannah. Of course people there are much frightened. I have been in a good many tight places in my life, but never saw anything to equal this. It was a common thing to see them bury ten before breakfast, and the same number before supper, and so we used to sit on deck and watch them carry the bodies along to their long home, day after day, and finally requested the authorities to remove the burial place, which was right in front of the ship. The sights we used to see were too much for the strongest of us. I hope it will be the last of that kind I shall see.[26]

The *San Salvador* was not the only steamship carrying troops who had been infected with cholera. Others, including the *Herman Livingston*, boarded troops from Hart's Island that July and transported them as far as New Orleans. By the time troops disembarked at Fort Jackson below the city, several men had fallen victim to what clearly was the Asiatic cholera. By the end of July the disease was rampant throughout both the regiment as well as the city itself; 247 cases were reported, with 143 deaths among the troops.[27] The disease was of course not confined to New Orleans; the city merely represented a focal point as troops were dispersed both west into Texas and north along the Mississippi. During August and September cholera was reported in western Kentucky, Nashville, Memphis, and then Cincinnati, all linked directly or indirectly to the initial outbreak on Governor's Island in New York; at least five medical officers died of the disease contracted while attending to victims. The post at Newport Barracks in Kentucky, across the river from Cincinnati, in particular was a point of origin for the epidemic in the Midwest. Troops from Governor's Island had arrived there in mid–July. The first victim was a woman who had accompanied the men on the trip. By the end of July over 100 cases had broken out among the troops. During the following months hundreds of the men were dispersed to sites elsewhere in Kentucky and Tennessee, some carrying the disease with them.

Cholera may have reached Detroit from several directions, no single one of which can be considered the specific point for the infection. On May 29, three children allegedly contracted and died of the disease after traveling from New York on the Great Western Railway, though some reports attributed the illness to "simple" dysentery. The fact that these victims, whether of cholera or something else, had been traveling by railroad was noteworthy for another reason. Prior to the war most travel between port cities such as Buffalo and Detroit had been by steamship. The extensive network of railroads that was developing throughout the country—including the transcontinental rail system now in place to the West Coast—meant carriers could disseminate throughout the region in a matter of days. The question of quarantining ports frequently appeared before boards of health, including those of Buffalo and Detroit. The conclusion was that such quarantines had been quickly becoming obsolete, given the ability to travel by rail between the cities, including Canadian cities.

At least one physician, a Dr. Lewis, had a new idea at this time as to the cause of the disease: "During the prevalence of the cholera in the West, the cases of the disease were much the most numerous on the shady side of the streets. He thinks that people who live in cellars are much more likely to take it than those whose dwellings are provided with good ventilation and plenty of sunlight."[28] While proper ventilation would certainly improve the quality of life, in itself it would do little to prevent the appearance of the disease. Once again the local newspaper, in advance of the impending epidemic, published advice, some of which was useful:

> Impure water and decaying articles of food must be avoided. The food must be strengthening, but always moderate. Intoxicating liquors must not be freely used. Intemperate persons must suffer severely from the disease. Keep the bowels warm, for which purpose use flannel bands. Ventilation of dwellings is of the utmost importance. We see how it is in overcrowded ships and jails, where the disease produces the most terrible havoc; and if persons who are infected with cholera in any place directly afterward go to live in foul air, they are likely to be seized with the full force of the disease, while those who go to healthy homes and pure air may suffer little or nothing at all from their exposure to the cholera poison in the infected districts. Therefore all dwellings should be thoroughly ventilated and cleansed when an epidemic comes. People must keep the doors and windows of their homes open, regardless of the weather, and protect themselves meanwhile by clothing. The common practice of putting chloride of lime in rooms when the air is corrupt is not a good substitute for ventilation.[29]

Brodie's proposal of the previous November that a city dispensary be established was also implemented that spring in Detroit. On April 12, a meeting of the incorporators of the Detroit City Dispensary Association was held in the office of the mayor. Fifteen prominent physicians and other notables of the city, including the omnipresent Zina Pitcher, were named trustees for one year, ending the following April 1. The purpose of the association was to "supersede the necessity of the office of city physicians."[30] More specifically, the specific duties of the association were

> to form a Medical Dispensary where the poor of our city can be provided with medicines gratuitously. Several physicians have already signified their willingness to donate their professional services for the use of those of that portion of our community who are unable to pay for medical attendance.... The expenses of the enterprise are expected to be borne partly from voluntary contributions. It is hoped that the Common Council will make a liberal appropriation which will go far to lessen the expenses.[31]

Any resident of the city, unless rendered ineligible "by reason of vicious or dissolute habits,"[32] would be eligible for the free medical care. Nonresidents with recommendations provided by members of the city council or members of the clergy would also be eligible. Any (male) adult who contributed $5 to the association — no small sum of money for a working man — would become a member for one year, and any person donating $50 would become a life member of the corporation.

Dr. Pitcher noted that since the function of the board of health was to oversee the health of the city, and to make recommendations deemed proper to promote cleanliness, the Sanitary Committee would recommend to the Common Council the establishment of public baths. The council was requested to find suitable locations or the baths, and to oversee their construction.[33] The council subsequently decided that rather than incurring the expense of land purchases and construction of expensive buildings, two sites would be located on rafts built in the river, with separate divided apartments available for men, women and younger boys.[34]

What became of the public bath idea as a means to promote cleanliness among the lower classes? At least in the immediate future, the answer was little. A year later the local media at least acknowledged the possible impetus for the project provided by the fear of cholera:

> Two years ago [1865] ... we pointed out that sea-bathing was too expensive to be within reach of those whose means are limited, and that some steps should therefore be taken by the proper authorities to enable our city-bound population to enjoy those baths which promote at the same time cleanliness and health. But though our proposition was seconded by the Board of Health, midsummer came and went, and another whole twelve months passed by without anything being done to provide Detroit with a place where its people could enjoy the trifling of bathing at a trifling expense....
>
> Now, we ask, what are our authorities about? The cholera may visit us before the summer is gone.... Experience has shown that wherever free public baths have been established and maintained, as long, at least, as there is any danger from the frightful pestilence, the effects were most surprising.[35]

Among the most comprehensive analyses in Detroit of cholera, its causes and treatment, was that by Dr. Alonzo Benjamin Palmer (1815–1887), a local physician and professor of pathology at the University of Michigan.[36] Palmer had been editor of the short-lived *Peninsular Journal of Medicine*, later serving as dean of the medical school at the University of Michigan. Drawing on his experience in the field, Palmer reviewed what he believed were the underlying causes of the disease, the "symptomatology and pathology," and the treatments available for the victim.

He began by acknowledging that the specific cause of cholera remained obscure while outlining what it was not. More specifically, that it was not associated with any alleged "electrical state," nor malaria, nor the presence or absence of ozone, thereby negating some of the more unusual theories. Given the understanding of disease in general, and cholera in particular, in 1866, Palmer's ideas were arguably prescient in his summary of the current knowledge.

> It seems difficult to avoid the conclusion that there is not only a specific and peculiar cause for the disease, but that such cause consists of a material poison.... If the poison be supposed to be an organism, whether vegetable or animal, the law of propagation will account for the increase.... The question of the contagiousness of cholera is one that has been much mooted, and it must be confessed, sometimes, without a clear appreciation of what constitutes a contagious disease. Strictly and properly defined, a contagious disease is one produced by a poison generated in the body of an individual affected by the same malady. Thus in small pox an animal poison is produced in the progress of the affection, which, when communicated by any means to one susceptible to its action, the same disease is reproduced.[37]

Palmer was correct in his assumption that the agent of cholera, though not a poison in the modern sense of the term, was capable of reproduction, and was indeed contagious in the sense that it would pass from person to person.

Once Palmer acknowledged the agent was capable of reproduction, he began to speculate on exactly where this was taking place — in the victim or in the environment:

> The facts in the history of cholera do not prove that this poison is exclusively produced in the bodies of the sick — but, on the contrary, in my judgment, they indicate that the poison is often, at least, produced independently of the bodies of those laboring under the disease, and that it is usually produced, multiplied and diffused independently of those affected by it.... I by no means affirm that the poison is to no extent, or in no degree produced in the sick, but it seems to me clearly that it is not wholly or chiefly so produced.[38]

Palmer was close in his understanding of the nature of the contagion, though again limited to the ideas of the times. The cholera bacillus, we now understand, can reproduce either within the human host (and then be disseminated through fecal contamination) or in an appropriate environment outside of the host. Palmer also addressed the prevailing prejudice that often blamed the victim in acquiring the disease:

> With regard to the classes of persons most liable in the same localities to be attacked, and become its victims, — the intemperate, the destitute, the filthy, the vicious, the enfeebled, the terrified, and the degraded, are immeasurably more subject to its ravages than those in opposite conditions. Yet when the poison is abundant and possesses great activity, no class or condition can claim an exemption.[39]
>
> The localities most liable to the spread of cholera, other things being equal, are low, moist, and particularly *filthy* [italics in original] situations. Warm climates and seasons are more favorable than cold, and a densely populated region more than one sparsely settled. It is more liable to follow water-courses and thoroughfares, partly because they are usually more low, filthy, and densely populated; and partly, no doubt, because the poison is conveyed by intercommunication.[40]

Palmer correctly understood the essential epidemiology of the disease, that it is likely associated with filth (sewage), is primarily a disease of warmer weather, and that it is somehow associated with a water supply.

Still, Palmer remained supportive of the theories of Max von Pettenkofer, briefly alluded to above, that while some form of fecal contamination or poison may be necessary for the disease to develop, it is nevertheless insufficient for the disease. "Predisposing or accessory causes" included decomposing matter in the host, resulting from the ingestion of putrescent food or water contaminated by sewage or similar matter, the "inspiration of air" contaminated with "miasmatic emanations," excessive exercise or injury, and/or insufficient supplies of air. The question of whether direct ingestion of sewage-contaminated water, in the absence of any miasma or putrescent material, led to contagion, was certainly on the mind of colleagues: "Is not the subsoil water the direct vehicle of the poison when, and only when, used for drinking purposes, as [John] Snow and [Charles] Richardson affirm? And is not the alleged necessity of interchange between the cholera germ and the soil an unnecessary incident in the propagation of cholera? i.e. would not the fresh excrement of a cholera patient admitted into the mouth, or inhaled, as in the act of washing dirty clothes, be enough to propagate the disease?"[41]

Palmer's methods for treatment were similar to those previously described by other physicians: a combination of opium, camphor, calomel and "sugar of milk," in combination with dry cupping over the abdomen, spine or stomach. Little that was new could be found here,

10. Epidemic of 1866

and reviews of his work were at best neutral, the primary criticism being that Palmer included his hypotheses concerning the causes and pathology of the disease as facts.

As summarized above, two factors certainly played a role in the spread of cholera during this period: the building of a national railroad network and the movement of army troops from the focal point of the outbreak in New York. During earlier epidemics, steamboats were the major mechanism by which cholera was disseminated, and these conveyances continued to play some role in 1866; outbreaks in both Savannah and New Orleans were the result of troop movements by water. But to a greater extent it was the railroads that provided a means for cholera to spread through the region: "Trains from the Eastern ports outstripped the steamboats to Cincinnati, Louisville, Chicago and St. Louis in carrying the seeds of the scourge, just as they were winning the race for the commerce, travel and romance of the upper interior valley."[42] That year over 50,000 persons in the United States were victims of the disease.

Detroit was spared during the summer of 1866, as sanitation and quarantine procedures instituted through the board of health were effective in preventing any significant outbreak of the disease. Other cities in the Midwest were not as fortunate. St. Louis suffered over 3,500 deaths due to cholera, and Chicago over 1,000. The total number of deaths in Detroit attributed to cholera for the year was fewer than 20, with 10 of the deaths occurring in the month of July. Even assuming the numbers represented a significant undercount — total deaths for the year were reported to be just over 1,300 — it was clear that a major outbreak had been averted.

While sporadic cases of cholera would continue to appear in Detroit in future decades, the year of 1866 represented the last time the disease appeared in anything approaching a significant number of cases.

11

The 1870s and Beyond

In 1873 an outbreak of cholera once again took place in the United States, the last such outbreak during the nineteenth century; the epidemic was largely confined to the Mississippi Valley. As had been the situation in previous outbreaks, the focal point of the infection was New Orleans. Steamboats ferrying passengers on the river brought the disease north to other ports along both the Mississippi and Ohio rivers. It was generally the deck-passengers, the poorest among the travelers, who would carry the disease. It was not unusual for the ship's captain to ignore or deny the existence of the disease, in part to avoid creating panic, and attribute the symptoms to the eating of green fruit or vegetables. Once passengers became ill, with vomiting and diarrhea, and contaminated clothing or freight — the victim did not always have the "luxury" of using the water closet — the disease would quickly spread throughout the vessel.

Chicago, with 116 deaths resulting from cholera, was the closest city to Detroit to suffer from the outbreak. By this time the epidemiology of the disease had become clear, even if the etiological agent had not yet been established. The epidemic was correctly attributed to situations in which the sanitary laws had not been followed. The total mortality for the 1873 outbreak was estimated at 7,350, with most occurring in Kentucky and Tennessee.

Only two deaths from cholera were reported in Michigan that year.[1] Ironically, the dearth of this disease in Detroit in 1873 led to squabbling among the city politicians and the board of health, centering on whether the board was even doing its job protecting the citizenry against disease or was merely allowing the aldermen who constituted the Board to draw an extra $1.50: "Alderman Woolly said the present board was a fraud and a humbug.... They get together four or five times a year to talk over the small-pox, frightening the people of the interior and driving them

11. The 1870s and Beyond

to other cities to purchase their merchandise. It would be some relief to take a good square turn at the Asiatic cholera."[2]

Despite the internecine arguments among the city administrators, the presence of cholera in port cities such as St. Louis, Nashville and Cincinnati, the same sites that in the past had served as focal points for spread of the disease into Detroit, raised legitimate concerns among members of the board of health. Once again the citizens of the city were reminded of the necessity for proper cleanliness and sanitation procedures:

> The city, instead of being absolutely beautiful and clean, is only a little more so than other cities, and falls far short of what it might be and ought to be. Too much reliance has been placed upon the city's natural advantages in this respect, and the people have fallen into the habit of neglecting the most ordinary precautions against disease. Every householder ought at this season of the year, if at no other, to make a thorough examination of his premises for the purpose of ascertaining whether he is holding out any inducements to fever or cholera. If he is, it is his most immediate and urgent duty to remove them. The public as a whole has also a duty to perform in this matter.... Let anyone who flatters himself that the city has extended no invitation to disease make a tour of the back streets and give an occasional glance at the alleys and vacant lots. Let him note the fragrance which emanates from barns and outbuildings [outhouses] and pools of stagnant water and then consult his physician as to the disease producing power of these agencies; and when he has done all these things let him look at the methods at present pursued for securing cleanliness and feel entirely free from apprehension if he can.[3]

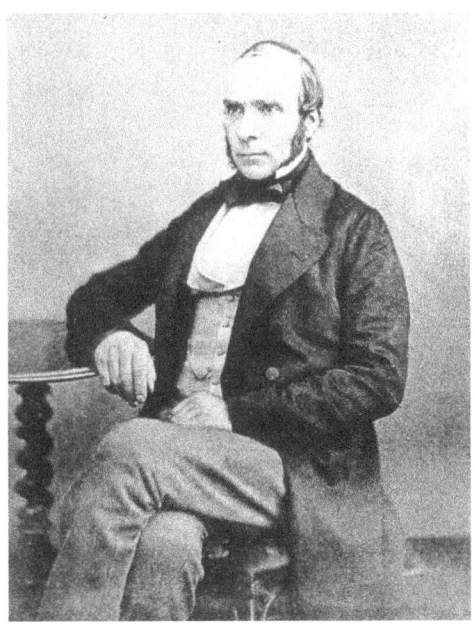

John Snow, English physician whose epidemiological studies of cholera outbreaks in London during the 1840s and 1850s helped establish the waterborne nature of the disease (image from the History of Medicine, National Library of Medicine).

165

The responsibilities of the individual vis-à-vis the health of the community at large, and the right of the government to require certain behaviors by the individual, remains a controversy even in the present day. Among the issues is the requirement of vaccinations for young children. Using a single example, should an individual child be required to receive the whooping cough vaccine even against the parents' wishes, or should parents be allowed to place the larger community at theoretical risk for an epidemic if the child is not immunized?

The sanitation system had also undergone significant change during the recent decades. The population of Detroit had more than doubled between 1840 (ca. 9100 persons) and 1850 (ca. 21,000). In the ensuing 20-plus years, the population had grown nearly five-fold (to more than 90,000 persons), clearly making the sanitation system that had been largely developed during the 1830s obsolete. Merely to keep the city supplied with pure water required the system to run 24 hours; any shutdown for repairs could render the city waterless. The system underwent significant expansion in 1849 with a new pump and engine that supplied much of the existing city; a new reservoir was also built near the present site of Eastern Market, approximately one mile northeast of the downtown.

In 1852 a board of trustees was established to oversee the system, with the power to carry out any legal acts necessary to maintain a proper function of the system. The board was transformed into the Board of Water Commissioners the following year. Among the first jobs was to construct a new reservoir; the new nine-million-gallon system was functioning by 1857. By 1871, 16 public drinking fountains had been set up. The inlet pipe to pump water into the city was lengthened into the river by another 160 feet. As the population continued to increase, reaching nearly 286,000 by the end of the century, the commission relocated the facilities farther upriver on Jefferson Avenue at what became known as Water Works Park, while modernizing the system even further. The park continues today, supplying over 240 million gallons of (now treated) water per day to the citizenry.

The Wayne County Medical Society, which had been established in 1866, once again proved unworkable. At its peak, the society had enrolled approximately 40 members. While the participants included physicians from the communities of Wyandotte and Wayne, the overwhelming

11. The 1870s and Beyond

majority in the membership were from the city of Detroit. Perhaps more important in determining the potential long-term success of the organization was the issue of advertising, a bane of previous medical societies. As the local media explained the tiff:

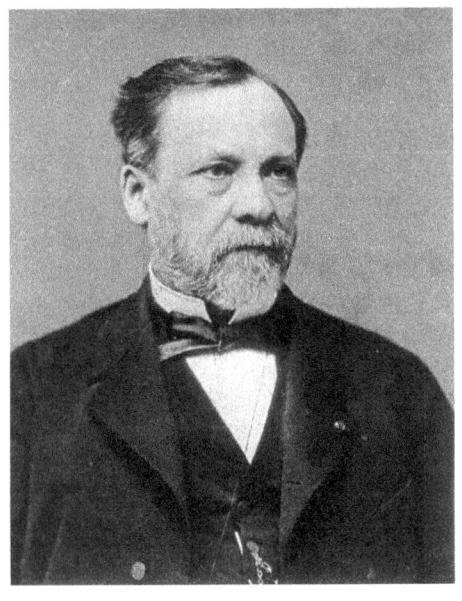

Louis Pasteur, French chemist who helped contribute to the germ theory of disease. His work included development of anthrax and rabies vaccines (image from the History of Medicine, National Library of Medicine).

> Some of the more aggressive spirits chafed under certain restrictions of the code and said and did things which the conservatives and high-toned sticklers sighed over and denounced as unprofessional and in violation of the ethical rules which had been laid down for their guidance. The most audacious, not to say unpardonable, of these so-called violations of professional etiquette, were various ingenious methods of "advertising" with which the aggressive members were charged. After a grave investigation withering resolutions of censure were passed. The snake was only scotched, however, and matters in the Society went on from bad to worse. A meeting of the Society was held last Thursday night, and after a long and heated discussion it was declared to be no longer fit to live.[4]

The demise of the society lasted a mere several weeks. The resurrection took place on August 17, with Dr. William Brodie, the previous president, resuming his role in that position, and a membership of some 20 physicians. Among the changes in the by-laws was the removal of any items not directly related to professional subjects, and allowing the board of directors to address these issues. The members apparently came to the conclusion that the function of the society, the dissemination of medical knowledge as well as providing advice for the health of the citizens of the county, was too important for the petty differences that had disrupted previous attempts to maintain a relationship among its members

Cholera in Detroit

to be the determining factors in success of the organization. Brodie served as president until his retirement in 1884. The society continued to evolve and continues in existence today.

It was not until 1881 that cholera again broke out in Detroit in significant numbers, claiming over 100 victims in July alone of that year, as well as smaller numbers of victims in the surrounding months. The disease had once again been widespread throughout the Midwest — affecting Chicago and Cincinnati among other major cities — and any one of these may have been the focal point into Detroit. Once again, however, the city was fortunate in that sanitation procedures set in motion in recent years, including attempts to ensure a safer water supply by extending the intake valve beyond any remaining sites of sewage contamination, limited the outbreak within the city and surrounding county. When a Detroit health officer, Dr. Orlando Williams Wight, was later queried as to how safe the city was from future outbreaks, the reply was,

> Now, in the city of Detroit, the water supply is beyond the reach of contamination. The intake is beyond the mouths of all sewers in the city. There are no towns on Lake St. Clair or on the river above large enough or near enough to pollute the great stream. No city in the United States has a water supply so secure from the contamination of cholera discharges as that of our city. It having been abundantly proved and it having been so declared by all the best authorities in the world that polluted drinking water is the most potent means of diffusing cholera, the conclusion is clear and inevitable that Detroit, so far as this most important of all factors is concerned,

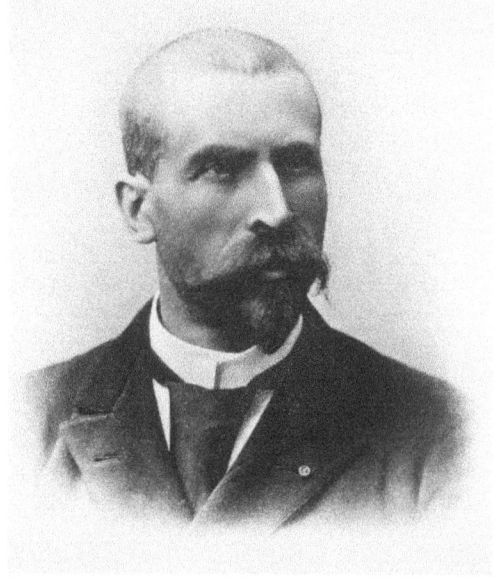

Émile Roux, French physician and colleague of Louis Pasteur who led the French Commission studying the cholera outbreak in Egypt during the 1880s (image from the History of Medicine, National Library of Medicine).

is especially secure against an epidemic of that dread disease.... Cholera is not contagious in the sense that smallpox, scarlet fever, measles diphtheria, and many other zymotic diseases are contagious. The germs of the infection are in the discharges of the patient. If these are cared for, with skill and energy, the battle is already half won.[5]

Wight was clearly cognizant by this time, 1884, that cholera is a "zymotic" infectious disease, one associated with a biological agent and not solely due to an esoteric atmospheric miasma. Was Wight aware that the germ of cholera had been identified? In his discussion he presented no evidence of being aware of Robert Koch's discovery and reporting of the actual etiological agent, which had taken place by that time. If Wight followed the medical reports, some presented in the local media earlier that year, it is highly unlikely he would have been completely ignorant of that latest information pertaining to cholera.

> The investigations made by the commission in Egypt last year had already indicated the existence in all true cases of cholera of a peculiar microscopic parasite, or bacillus, as it is termed in medical language. In all cases which came under their examination, Dr. Koch and his colleagues observed these parasites in great number, both in the intestines of the persons who had died of cholera and in the dejecta of cholera patients. The same parasites were uniformly found in all cholera cases examined in India. Moreover, although looked for with minuteness and care, no parasites corresponding to them could be found in connection with other diseases, such as dysentery and diarrhea, which have some resemblance to cholera. The fact, therefore, between the close relation between the parasite and the disease of cholera would seem to be placed beyond a doubt. The coincidence would not in itself, however, as is obvious, warrant us in regarding the parasite as the cause of the malady; it may be the consequence.
>
> From a further discovery made by the commission in Calcutta, there is no reason to believe that the relation of parasite to disease is one of cause [i.e., the disease mah have preceded the presence of the parasite]; in short that the parasite is the long sought for cholera germ. While the commission was in Calcutta a sporadic outbreak of cholera of great intensity occurred in the native quarter of the town, in the neighborhood of a dirty tank or pond. On examining the water in this pond, Dr. Koch and his colleagues discovered to their joy that it swarmed with the parasite which they had hitherto failed to find outside the human subject. The water had been used, according to Indian habits, both for drinking and bathing purposes by the people among whom the outbreak had occurred. It was further observed that as the outbreak subsided the water became clear of the parasite.... But the last link in completing the chain of evidence has yet to be forged. All the attempts of Dr.

Koch and his colleagues to artificially propagate cholera by means of the parasite, whether found in the water or in the human subject, have been without success. Many experiments have been made with a view to reproduce the disease by inoculation in animals, but all have failed.[6]

A more complete description of Koch and the role of the German Commission in isolating the etiological agent of cholera is provided in the following chapter. But here the anonymous writer, obviously versed in the science of bacteriology, has summarized the process by which the cholera bacillus was identified: its presence at the site of infection, the intestine of the human victim, and the means by which the "parasite" was encountered, in the drinking water. The presence of the bacillus in the water preceding the infection was critical in demonstrating which came first—the disease, or the growth of the parasite. The writer also noted a major difficulty encountered by Koch in demonstrating the ability of the bacillus to produce the disease, cholera does not develop in most non-human test animals.

In addition to cholera, by 1884 several other important human diseases had been shown to result from infections by specific agents—most notably tuberculosis (again by Koch)—and it would require no stretch of imagination by Wight, whether or not he was aware of Koch's work, to assume cholera was also such a disease. Wight also (correctly) pointed out the means of transmission, through the "discharges of the patient." By implication he pointed out that in this manner cholera differed from other infectious diseases that could be transmitted readily from person to person. Wight later noted the precautions that medical attendants would take in examining patients, carrying disinfectants for use on their persons or in treating diarrheal discharges. In the past, cholera patients had been placed in quarantine, often in pest-houses established for that purpose. Since in the absence of direct contact with the patient the disease would not be transmitted, there was no need for establishing this form of medical station. Patients could remain in their homes, or if the patient was too poor to have such a residence, tents could be placed in open areas—this being the period of warm weather—for treatment and care. Wight was particularly emphatic when asked about the efficacy of cordoning off areas in order to prevent interaction with travelers from cholera-infested areas, or in exposing travelers to large amounts of disinfectants, as had been done in earlier cholera epidemics in Detroit:

11. The 1870s and Beyond

"Fumigating travelers ... is simply ridiculous. Cholera germs are carried in the intestines beyond the reach of fumigations."[7]

The decade of the 1880s saw the beginning and spread of what subsequently became recognized as the fifth cholera pandemic, once again originating in the Bengal region of India and spreading throughout Asia and the Middle East. As we shall see, it was during this outbreak in Egypt and India that the etiological agent was finally isolated. The well-founded fear that once again cholera would enter the United States, and more specifically, given the central role in immigration played by Detroit, develop into epidemic proportions in Michigan, led the governor of the state, Josiah Begole, to propose prophylactic measures to protect the state. In a report to the legislature early in 1885 entitled "Danger from Cholera," Begole pointed out,

> Cholera has never prevailed as extensively in Europe as during the last few months without sooner or later coming to the United States. From our situation on the great lines of travel and of immigration [most notably the lake cities of Port Huron and Detroit], Michigan is especially liable to receive infected persons or infected baggage. Our local boards of health are authorized to make such regulations as they may deem necessary for the public health and safety, respecting any articles which are capable of containing or conveying any infection or contagion, or of creating any sickness, when such articles shall be brought into, or conveyed from, their township, or into or from any vessel.... The cities of Port Huron or Detroit can hardly be asked to bear the expense of such an inspection of the thousands of immigrants annually entering the country at these

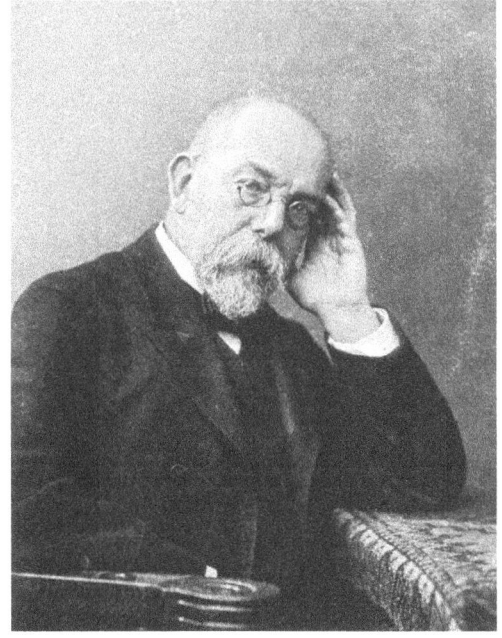

Robert Koch, German physician who in 1884 identified the etiological agent of cholera (image from the History of Medicine, National Library of Medicine).

Cholera in Detroit

cities.... In view of the danger from cholera, I would recommend an appropriation for an epidemic contingent fund, to be used in the discretion of the Governor, under the direction of the State Board of Health, for the prevention or suppression of outbreaks of cholera, should the danger become imminent and a necessity arise for the use of said fund or any part of it.[8]

The act was signed into law by the incoming governor, Russell Alger, in June of that year; however, it would not go into effect until September. The act allocated up to $10,000 to be used by the state board of health. While fear of an outbreak of cholera was one of the major driving forces in the approval by the legislature, the allocation could as easily be applied to any other infectious disease (e.g., smallpox) that might be threatening. In fact, smallpox had recently broken out in Montreal and several other Canadian cities at this time (July 1885), and as a legislator pointed out, "There can be no doubt but for this new danger [smallpox] the legislature would have struck out the words 'or other communicable diseases,' making the Act of no use except for the prevention of the introduction of cholera."[9]

It was not the presence (albeit decreased) of cholera in Europe, or even in New York, which was of the greater concern, at least in Wight's mind. Cholera was now endemic to the Western Hemisphere:

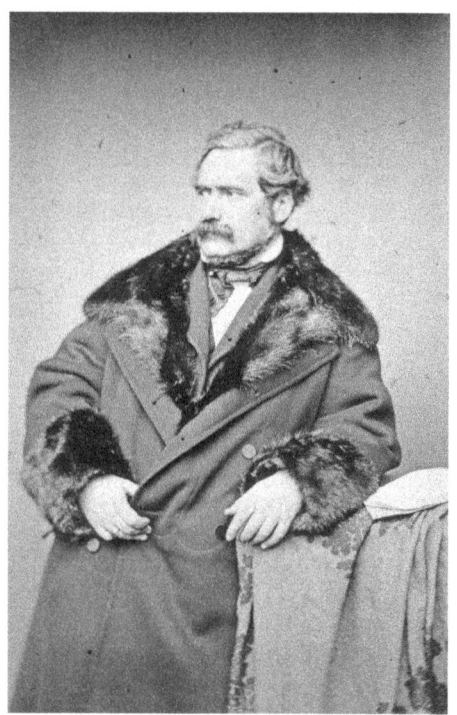

Max von Pettenkofer, German chemist and hygienist whose miasmatic theory of cholera was in contradiction to Koch's theory of contagion (image from the History of Medicine, National Library of Medicine).

> Seasoned sanitarians apprehend transmission of cholera from Spain to Cuba and from Cuba to the Gulf Coast of the United States. Such transmission may be quite rapid. The foulness of West India cities will promote the swift growth of the disease,

and fugitives from it are likely enough to escape with its contagion to the United States. Quarantine on the gulf is now quite effective, and the danger in that direction is much less than it was a few years ago. There are very few Spanish immigrants to this country. Consequently the danger to this country is much less than it would be if Germany or Great Britain were infected. There is really less danger for this reason than there was last year when the cholera raged in France and Italy.... No pains have been spared to put Detroit in a condition to meet its advent. The city is really cleaner at the present time than it has ever been before.[10]

12

Isolation and Identification of the Cholera Bacillus

Between the beginning of the first cholera pandemic in 1817 and the end of the nineteenth century, five major cholera pandemics spread throughout Europe and the Middle East. The Atlantic Ocean proved to be merely a temporary barrier, as either immigration from Europe or other forms of travel brought the disease to North America. As described earlier, in 1832 the disease spread from Buffalo to Detroit, and eventually passed through what is now the midwestern United States. Estimates of total mortality in America during the nineteenth century vary, but unquestionably reached well into the hundreds of thousands. Detroit suffered several major outbreaks until the role played by contaminated water supplies was established and public health became more formalized.

The cause of the disease remained a mystery through much of the nineteenth century. As we shall see, even after what we now know is the etiological agent, a small curved bacterium named *Vibrio cholerae*, had been isolated, the role of this organism in the disease remained controversial. On one side were the "contagionists," those who believed cholera was an infection resulting from ingestion of contaminated water, while opposing them in thought were the "miasmatists," physicians who believed the disease arose endemically from the release of vapors from contaminated soil. Eminent medical personnel could be found on either side of the argument even as late as the first decade of the twentieth century.

Two classical epidemiological studies of cholera outbreaks in London during the 1850s by British physician John Snow (1813–1858) were among the earliest such works to significantly contribute to understanding the source of the disease. Nevertheless, an acceptance of the role

12. Isolation and Identification of the Cholera Bacillus

played by an infectious agent would not come to pass until decades after Snow's death.

Snow was well known in England for reasons beyond his study of cholera. He is considered among the earliest pioneers in the use of ether or chloroform as an anesthetic, even administering the vapors to Queen Victoria during the birth of the last two of her nine children during the mid–1850s. The success of what at the time was still considered a highly controversial practice, even by authors for the medical journal *The Lancet*—this was, after all, the queen—firmly established the young surgeon as a significant figure in British medicine. Victoria was not the first patient on whom Snow used ether or chloroform as an anesthetic; he had published several monographs on the subject some years earlier. But the work did lend an aura of credibility to his later work with cholera.[1]

The prevailing theory was that some form of miasma emanating from soil or water, the odor of putrefaction as an example, was the basis for the disease. This was by far the most popular contemporary view of the cause, and one espoused even by the London sanitation commissioner, Edwin Chadwick. Snow was convinced otherwise. His hypothesis was that the origin of cholera involved a contagion of some sort, an idea that began with the outcome of his observation of the 1848 outbreak in London, one that ultimately claimed over 14,000 lives. Snow began his treatise on the epidemiology of the London epidemics by describing the role of a German seaman, John Harnold, as a point source of the outbreak.[2] Harnold was a member of the crew on the steamer ship *Elbe*, which had previously been docked in Hamburg during the time of a cholera outbreak in that German city. Following a brief passage from the German city, followed by the docking of the steamer in London, Harnold disembarked from the ship and lodged in a house on Gainsford Street in Horsleydown, then a small parish on the river Thames and now part of London. Harnold developed a clear case of cholera on September 22, dying within hours. Several days later a man named Blenkinsopp, whose first name appears lost to history, lodged in the same room in which Harnold had died, and subsequently developed cholera as well. Blenkinsopp, who presumably succumbed to the disease, though Snow does not indicate such, was attended by the same physician who had previously seen Harnold. Snow felt the presence of two cases of cholera originating in the same room could not be a coincidence; nor could the presence of vapors account for the rapidly developing symptoms of cholera on the same day Harnold rented the room. Reports from other sources in Scotland and elsewhere that described outbreaks of cholera coincident with the presence of ships on which outbreaks had taken place further convinced Snow of a role played by some type of contagion.

Two epidemiological studies solidified the role of water contamination as the source for the cholera outbreak. Once the 1848 outbreak had run its course, cholera did not again appear in London for some five years. At the time, two of the companies that supplied water for portions of the city of London were the Lambeth Company and Southwark and Vauxhall Company. The water from which Lambeth drew its supply had been changed from the tidal region of the Thames to the cleaner Thames Ditton site in 1852; Southwark and Vauxhall continued to obtain their water from Battersea, located on the south side of the Thames, an area that included the tidal region, and that was subject to sewage discards from any shipping fleet dumping its ballast or sewage into the river. Cholera had broken out on one of the ships from the Baltic fleet earlier in the summer, the likely source of the outbreak investigated by Snow. Comparing the incidence of cholera among persons in the same region of London, differing only by which of the two companies supplied the water, Snow observed a difference of nearly ten-fold in households obtaining water from Lambeth Company as compared with those households obtaining water from Southwark and Vauxhall, the latter exhibiting the much greater incidence.[3] Snow's belief was that the water contaminated by the presence of the disease on the ship, specifically the sewage dumped into the Thames, was the source of this outbreak.

Snow's second study, often referred to as that of the "Broad Street pump," involved the investigation of an epidemic of cholera that took place in London during the summer of 1854. Utilizing a spot map to note the sites or households in which the disease had occurred, Snow observed that nearly all persons who developed cholera had either directly or indirectly — as in the case of a bar located some distance from the pump — obtained their water from that pump.[4]

A myth grew from the story that Snow convinced the authorities to remove the pump handle, after which the incidence of new cases

12. Isolation and Identification of the Cholera Bacillus

immediately declined.[5] In fact the numbers of new cases had already begun a decline prior to the removal of the handle, a fact even noted by Snow in the pamphlet that he subsequently published describing the work.[6] Still, Snow was correct in his premise that the pump was the focal point for the outbreak.

Snow also pointed out the presence of flocculent material in the contaminated pump water, though the presence was attributed to the "decomposition of other matter."[7] Despite Snow's publication of his two works, one smaller description of the 1848 outbreak and then a more complete treatise six years later, both were largely forgotten outside of England in the decades after his early death from a stroke. Robert Koch, who subsequently identified the bacillus as the etiological agent of cholera, even failed to make reference to the earlier works by Snow. It was only in the initial years of the next century that Snow's contributions became more generally acknowledged, even to the extent of becoming a standard "read" in any course on epidemiology.[8]

The actual discovery of the cholera bacillus, and more importantly its role as the etiological agent of the disease, became mired in the issue of prior discovery, as well in as the politics and nationalism of the times. It is important to remember that what became known as the germ theory of disease, the knowledge that illness was associated with a specific infectious agent that could be transmitted through a variety of mechanisms, only became accepted in the period of the 1870s and beyond; indeed the period between roughly the 1870s and the new century is often referred to as the Golden Age of Microbiology, reflecting the discovery of numerous infectious entities that were the etiological agents of specific diseases. Robert Koch (1843–1910), a German physician, and Louis Pasteur (1822–1895), a French chemist, are the two most celebrated figures for this era. Their roles represented a microcosm of the German and French nationalism that underlay much of their scientific work: "for the glory of France," or "for the glory of Germany," phrases used in a variety of contexts both before Pasteur and Koch, and long afterwards, perfectly summed up the respective nationalistic viewpoints of these scientific opponents. Their respective contributions were often placed in that context; France and Germany were frequently in opposition, both in the laboratory and, literally, on the battlefield.

There were additional challenges faced by physicians and scientists outside of Europe during this period. Among the most important was the perception that the most important scientific research was that which was carried out by German scientists. This research could be carried out in Germany itself, in the German states that preceded unification by Chancellor Otto von Bismarck in the 1870s, or in cities such as Vienna, the capital of Austria-Hungary. Despite the excellent work carried out in England and other European countries—the United States was largely a backwater during this period—the perception had a strong element of truth.[9] The most outstanding science, the most important discoveries, took place on the European continent.

So whom should we credit with the identification of a specific microorganism as the cause of cholera? With the passage of time and history historians have acknowledged the honor should probably fall to the Italian scientist Filippo Pacini (1812–1883).[10] Pacini has been most noted for his discovery of Pacinin corpuscles, capsular wrapped nerve endings in the skin that respond to pressure. In 1854, however, while studying the intestinal mucosa of patients who had died from cholera, Pacini observed curved or comma-shaped bacteria in histological specimens. The common feature he observed among most of these patients was the presence of the same microscopic organism, and Pacini suggested these might actually be the agents of the disease. Pacini did publish his findings that year (1854),[11] and followed this initial work with further publications in later years. Pacini correctly described the nature of the disease as a "massive loss of fluid and electrolytes due to a purely local action of the vibrio on the intestinal mucosa, and recommending in extreme cases the intravenous injection of ... sodium chloride [salt] in a liter of water."[12] Few contemporary physicians or scientists were aware of Pacini's observations, published in a language few read, and describing what appeared to be a localized outbreak in Florence. Posthumous recognition did eventually come to Pacini, as the International Committee on Bacteriological Nomenclature, a modern body that routinely oversees or recommends the naming of micro-organisms, recommended that the etiological agent for cholera should be named *Vibrio cholerae* Pacini 1854, an honor bestowed 82 years after Pacini's death.[13] There is no evidence that Koch was aware of Pacini's work when he subsequently described his own re-discovery of the cholera bacillus a year after Pacini's death.

12. Isolation and Identification of the Cholera Bacillus

Koch's contribution to the cholera story began in Egypt. Though the first pandemic of the disease began about 1817 in India, cholera did not reach Egypt until 1831, when an estimated 5 percent of the population may have died from the disease — approximately 150,000 victims.[14] The threat from cholera, and waterborne diseases in general, only increased in the following decades as land and irrigation reforms, carried out in order to enable the Egyptian economy to compete with those in the West, resulted in greater risk of contamination of drinking water with human excrement. As described by contemporary observers, "Cairo was a city of cesspools that flooded and spread filth at high Nile, or dried up and left human waste to blow in the wind at low Nile."[15]

Several additional factors proved significant by the time cholera made another appearance in Egypt during the early 1880s. First, the Suez Canal was opened for traffic during the fall of 1869, eliminating the need for shipping between Europe and Asia — particularly from the British colony of India — to travel around the coast of Africa. The canal was initially overseen by the Suez Canal Authority of Egypt. But financial crises during the ensuing years resulted in Egypt's rulers selling a majority share of the canal to England. Political turmoil and resentment among much of the population against European encroachment on Egyptian autonomy reached a critical point by the end of the decade, terminating in rioting in parts of the country. During the late summer of 1882, British troops occupied several cities in the country, suppressing the rioting and effectively making Egypt into another British colony.

The result was that when cholera appeared in Mecca in 1881, despite measures instituted by the International Quarantine Board in Alexandria to contain the disease, it quickly spread into Egypt; whether at first across the Suez Canal, or into Damietta at the site where the Nile enters the Mediterranean Sea, is uncertain. Between June 1883, when it first appeared in that port city, and the end of the year, cholera killed an estimated 58,000 persons. Even the British troops stationed in Egypt suffered from the outbreak, with 139 deaths, representing a mortality rate of over 70 percent.[16] If nothing else, the threat to the British catalyzed action on their part to address the problem of a contaminated water supply. England was even accused by Germany of being the source of the epidemic, with cholera being carried on those British ships that entered the canal after traveling from India.[17]

Concern grew among the European powers, most notably England, France and Germany, that the outbreak might yet spread to the European continent, a fear well founded in precedent. The result was that each of the three countries, for their own political and scientific reasons, decided to send commissions to determine the source of the latest outbreak. There was also the underlying desire to identify the etiological agent, assuming the disease was caused by an infectious entity.

British Commission

The British Commission arrived first, establishing a laboratory in Cairo in July 1883 with Surgeon-General William Guyer Hunter (1829– 1902), newly returned from India, in charge, and a total of ten physicians. The British investigators were hampered by several factors. First, they were working on a limited budget, and their equipment consisted largely of microscopes for examining water. To their credit, the physicians who composed the commission visited a number of infected villages, interviewing local doctors and maintaining careful records. Even so, the greater handicap was the preconceived notion among British physicians that cholera was associated with miasmas and was not some form of contagion. The belief was more than simply a scientific notion, but encroached on the political issue of the British role in the occupation of Egypt. If cholera had a local Egyptian origin rather than being a disease imported from India, England could not be held responsible. The conclusion of the British Commission was, "Facts ... lead to the conclusion that cholera, be it called by whatever name it may, has existed in Egypt for some time past."[18] In his final report to Earl Granville, secretary of state for foreign affairs, dated December 11, 1883, Hunter described the sanitary conditions of Alexandria, Egypt, as "deplorable": "There are no public latrines. A portion of the city only is sewered, and the sewers are unventilated. To windward of the city, thirteen public sewers, exclusive of many private drain-pipes, are constantly discharging their contents on the beach of a tideless sea. The house connections of the privies with the sewers are free.... The sulphurous gasses, the products of the combustion, readily found an entrance into the houses and created much alarm among the residents."[19]

12. Isolation and Identification of the Cholera Bacillus

In this manner Hunter laid the groundwork for his argument that conditions in the atmosphere were appropriate for development of the disease. He went on in the report to negate any role of an infectious agent as the cause of the disease:

> A cholera-germ is supposed to be a microscopic organism, capable of being imported from the country of its birth and that on being so imported in a country, provided a suitable soil-condition or conditions exist, it will develop and propagate itself, and from time to time manifest its presence by outbreaks of the disease.... The more advanced advocates of this theory state, moreover, that fresh outbreaks in European countries require for their populations fresh importation of germs from India, as the soil of Europe is not propitious to their cultivation and existence. They consequently always look for fresh importation of cases from India to account for any epidemic visiting a country, and refuse to accept evidence of the existence of the disease unless it can be so traced. A germ has never yet been proved to exist in connection with cholera. Its existence is assumed, partly because certain micro-organisms have been found in connection with certain maladies of an infectious or contagious character, and which have been pronounced by those who lend support to the germ-theory of disease [i.e., Koch, a German, and Pasteur, a Frenchman] to stand in a causal relation to them."[20]

Hunter went on to cite the observations of two colleagues: "The investigations of Dr. Timothy Lewis and Dr. Douglas Cunningham did not afford any evidence in favor of the existence of a specific poison contained in cholera-excrete peculiar to them alone, and giving rise to special phenomena.[21] ... The German mission, at the head of which is Dr. [Robert] Koch, is said, on the other hand, to have been more successful; and to have discovered the cholera-germ, a bacteroid body, having a rod or stave-like formation, and consequently a bacillus." Hunter followed with the disclaimer: "Dr. Koch, however, in his report ... is much more cautious in his remarks, and definitely states that he looks upon the experiments hitherto conducted as merely of an initiatory character, and expressly states that it is not to be assumed that these micro-organisms are the actual causes of the disease."[22]

These conclusions were also presented by Hunter when he spoke in January 1884 before the prestigious London Epidemiological Society. The society, among the first professional organizations devoted to the study of epidemiology, ironically had been founded in part by John Snow in 1850, by then the forgotten man in the study of cholera. Hunter restated his argument that cholera was an endemic disease in India, likely associated with the miasmas of putrefaction of the raw sewage routinely dumped into the food or water supply. Further contributing to the outbreak were the unusual weather patterns, which "reactivated" the cholera poison present in the soil.[23] The clear implication of course, was that the disease was not introduced from ships plying the Suez Canal, and that Britain had nothing to do with the current outbreak. Hunter was awarded with the honor of Knight Commander of the Order of St. Michael and St. George for the work of the commission and for absolving Britain of any responsibility in causing the epidemic.[24]

French Commission

The French Commission arrived on the heels of the departure of the British, in August 1883. The group of physicians was organized by the French government and was established with the guidance of Louis Pasteur. The commission included several of Pasteur's colleagues: Drs. Isidore Strauss (1845–1896), professor of medicine at the University of Paris, Émile Roux (1853–1933), Edmond Nocard (1850–1903), a professor of veterinary medicine, and Louis Thuiller (1856–1883). The aging Pasteur himself was not on site, and the commission was led by Roux.[25] Unlike the British Commission, the French were not hampered by as limited a budget; the French Chamber of Deputies and Senate had allotted 50,000 francs. However, by the time they established their laboratory, establishing their headquarters in the *Hopital Europèen* in Alexandria, the current epidemic had largely been spent, and relatively few cholera victims were available to study.

The commission did manage to carry out microscopic examination of intestinal contents during 24 autopsies, as well as microscopically observing the rice-water stools and vomitus from patients. The members also attempted to induce cholera in a variety of laboratory animals (guinea pigs, rabbits and mice, among others) by introducing stools obtained from cholera victims through a catheter into the alimentary tracts of the animals.[26] While there is no evidence any of the animals enjoyed the experience, none contracted cholera.

With lack of success either in identifying an infectious agent or in transmitting the disease to a laboratory animal — unknown at the time was that few non-human animals are susceptible to cholera—several members of the commission, Nocard and Thuiller, began in mid–September the studying of oxen that had recently died during an outbreak of cattle plague.[27] On the night and early morning of the 17th and 18th Thullier awoke with severe diarrhea, shortly afterwards collapsing. Despite measures to treat what was clearly cholera—iced champagne and subcutaneous injections of ether, neither of which would have been beneficial—Thullier died on the morning of the 19th.[28] When Thullier had been exposed is difficult to surmise as it had been over two weeks since the team had examined excreta from cholera victims. Thullier had also been previously warned by Pasteur of the dangerous nature of the assignment. There is no reason to think the warning had gone unheeded, and when or how Thullier became infected remains a mystery.

Despite the competition between Koch and Pasteur's teams, Koch and several German colleagues attended Thullier's funeral in Alexandria, which was held the afternoon of his death, and even provided two wreaths, which were attached to the coffin; Koch also served as one of the pallbearers for the coffin. Pasteur himself, unable to attend the funeral because of age and distance, was overcome with grief at the loss of his colleague and friend. The respect shown by Koch and his German colleagues, despite the nationalistic rivalry, at least provided a small measure of solace.

The three surviving members of the French Commission returned home in October following Thullier's death. In November the members of the commission presented an account of their findings before the Societe de Biologie in Paris. In describing the micro-organisms they had observed, they reported, "It is evident that, in the presence of such a great variety of organisms, it is impossible to single out and designate the one that, any more than another, might be the cause of cholera."[29] The small particles that had been observed by the members of the commission in blood of patients, and the source of the particles in the Thullier myth described in the endnote, were likely blood platelets.

German Commission

Once the establishment of the French Commission had been announced it appears that Berlin quickly set in motion the establishment of one of its own; the German Commission was authorized on August 9 and a week later was prepared to leave for Egypt, departing on August 20 for Port Said. The German Commission, which arrived in Alexandria four days later, on August 24, was composed of Robert Koch, the head of the commission, Georg Gaffky (1850–1918), Bernhard Fischer (1852–1915) and chemist Hermann Julius Paul Treskow. Since the French (and Italians, who were also present) had already occupied Egyptian facilities, the Germans were housed in the Greek hospital. Within a month the commission provided its first report: the members had observed specimens obtained from 12 patients as well as from autopsy material from ten victims of the disease. No microbes were observed in internal organs, while only a few microbes were observed in the vomitus. However, a large number of unusual microbes were observed in the intestinal contents from patients or victims, including a "specific type of bacterium found in the wall of the small intestine in cholera victims, but not in those who had died from other causes ... therefore be no doubt that they, the bacteria, stand in some relation to the cholera process." Koch was hesitant, however, to identify the bacteria he had observed as being the etiological agents of the disease:

> It is not to be concluded from the association with the latter with the presence of the bacilli in the intestinal mucosa that the bacilli are the cause of cholera. It could be the other way around, and it could equally well be that the cholera process results in such a disruption of the intestinal mucosa that the infiltration into the tissue of the intestinal mucosa of a particular kind of bacillus ... is made possible.... Whether the infection process or whether the bacterial invasion is primary, can be determined only by attempts to isolate the bacteria from the diseased tissues, grow them in pure cultures, and reproduce the disease by experimental infections in animals [which included fifty mice he had brought with him, as well as attempts to directly infect experimental animals *per rectum*].[30]

The caveat expressed by Koch represents one of the more important contributions to medical science by that German physician: Koch's Postulates. The Postulates represent the scientific procedure by which a specific organism may be linked to a disease: isolating and growing the organism in pure culture; inoculating a test animal and causing the disease; and finally reisolating the same organism from the test animal. Koch pointed out they were not able to reproduce cholera in test animals, a problem noted earlier that had been encountered by the French; as we

12. Isolation and Identification of the Cholera Bacillus

now are aware, the cholera bacillus does not cause the disease in most non-human animals.

By the fall of 1883 the number of new cases of cholera had significantly fallen in Egypt. Unable to provide proof for his belief that the "comma bacillus" he had observed was the agent of the disease, Koch requested permission from the British to continue their investigation in India where a fresh outbreak of the disease had taken place.

The Germans left Egypt in mid-November and arrived in Calcutta on December 11, Koch's fortieth birthday, after a voyage of some four weeks.[31] The British authorities in India, proved highly accommodating, perhaps surprising given the nature of the investigation; an identification of an infectious agent could easily implicate the British as the source of the earlier outbreak in Egypt. Among those who greeted Koch was Dr. James McNabb Cuningham (1829–1905), surgeon-general and sanitary commissioner for India, whose opinions would later differ sharply with Koch's conclusions on the contagious nature of cholera.[32] The Germans were given ready access to the medical facilities at the Medical College Hospital and to the laboratory building next to the hospital where large windows provided the light necessary for the microscopes of the time, and blinds to limit the sunlight when the room had to be kept cool.[33]

In a series of seven reports sent from Calcutta to Berlin between September 17, the day of Thullier's death, and March 4, 1884, just prior to his return to Berlin, Koch outlined the procedures he used in tracking the elusive cholera bacillus and finally defining its role as the agent of the disease. By necessity this was indirect. In attempting to follow Koch's Postulates, outlined above, Koch would have had to infect an experimental animal and re-isolate the organism; this proved impossible. Instead the question Koch posed was "whether these bacilli are normal inhabitants of the intestine, *or whether they occur exclusively in the intestines of cholera patients* and not in patients suffering from other forms of diarrhea such as dysentery"[34] [italics added]. Koch also noted that the incidence of new cases of cholera had fallen to less than a third of what had been the case earlier in the year, a change he ascribed to the "introduction of piped water supplies."[35] The implication was clear, and reminiscent of that expressed by John Snow more than 30 years earlier, that the source of the disease was in the contaminated water. The difference in the observations by Koch in 1884 from those by Snow in 1854 was that Koch had actually identified a specific micro-organism. Koch also addressed the difficulty in finding an experimental animal by rhetorically asking whether this would even be possible: "Were there a susceptible species, one would expect to find it in Bengal, where cholera exists throughout the year, but no animal infections have ever been seen. The proof afforded by the facts already cited 'is not weakened by the failure of the animal experiments.' The same was true of other infectious diseases, such as typhoid and leprosy."[36]

Koch's sixth report laid out the argument for the bacillus he observed as being the actual etiological agent. While in India the members of the commission had ultimately examined 92 victims: 52 autopsies and 40 live patients. The bacillus, which he described as a slightly curved, comma-shaped organism, was not straight like other bacilli and was therefore unique to the disease: it was observed only in cholera patients and only at the site of infection, the intestine, and not in the vomitus. The organism was so abundant in the rice-water diarrhea from these patients that "it was almost like a pure culture." Further, as the patient recovered the organism disappeared from the stools. Koch's logical conclusion, which he presented in his report, and then directly at the Conference for the Discussion of the Cholera Question on July 26, 1884, in Berlin, was that the described bacillus was the agent of the disease.[37]

The commission's presentation stimulated a heated discussion for several hours, but in the end there was little opposition, at least among those present, with the conclusion; among those present was Rudolph Virchow (1821–1902), considered among the most important of the German pathologists and an earlier skeptic regarding Koch's theory. While Virchow urged Koch to be careful since absolute proof was still lacking (in the form of an animal infection), he had no significant argument with the conclusions. Georg Gaffky, a member of the commission, described the role of a toxin that acted directly on the intestinal wall, a feature now known to be largely correct. (Koch also suggested the toxin might attack the cardiovascular system as well, which was incorrect.) The members of the commission were richly rewarded, receiving a grant from the Reichstag of 100,000 marks in gold, medals from Kaiser Wilhelm I, and praise from Chancellor Bismarck.[38] Koch also received from the crown prince, later Wilhelm II, the Order of the Throne with Star.[39]

Among those conspicuous by his absence was Dr. Max von Pettenkofer (1818–1901), earlier the chairman of the Imperial Cholera Commission and considered among the foremost experts in the study of cholera; his absence was even more noteworthy in that Koch and the other members of his commission had paid a courtesy visit to Pettenkofer in Munich prior to attending the conference.

Pettenkofer had earned a reputation as a research genius during his many years in the scientific field, with contributions in chemistry, in the art world — he once identified the cause of a haze that developed on paintings hung in galleries as a reaction in the varnish, and developed a method of treatment — and of course his role in medicine. When Koch announced his findings in 1884 pertaining to cholera, Pettenkofer had already spent much of his life in the study of the disease.[40]

Pettenkofer's hypothesis regarding the cause of cholera was sometimes referred to as the ground water theory. He believed an outbreak was associated with three environmental factors which he termed x, y and z. Pettenkofer considered the "x" to possibly be a germ "disseminated by human hands," the "y" factor "something which depends on place or time, the local disposition, including the quality or wetness of the soil"; and "z" the "individual disposition met with in all infectious diseases."[41] By 1892 Pettenkofer had conceded a role for the comma bacillus isolated by Koch, but continued to argue that by itself the organism was not sufficient to cause the disease. Pettenkofer's argument was based upon his own epidemiological observations: "There are not only cholera-immune people, but also cholera-immune places, and that even in places where cholera has prevailed there are seasons when it will not spread, although introduced."[42] The problem was the soil, not the organism. This was not to say that impure water did not create its own problems: "I myself am a drinking water fanatic but not so much for fear of typhoid fever or cholera. Impure water ... could disturb physiological processes in the human body and thus make the individual more susceptible to cholera."[43]

Pettenkofer paid more than mere lip service to his arguments against the role of the Koch bacillus; in a time-honored fashion carried out among many scientists, he tested this on himself:

> I had received from Hamburg, through my colleague, Dr. [Georg] Gaffky, a pure agar culture, and from this my junior colleagues, Drs. [Richard Friedrich] Pfeiffer[44] (1858–1945) and Eisenlohr, prepared a sufficient quantity of broth culture to be taken by the mouth.... One cubic centimeter of this was found to contain innumerable bacilli, after being diluted a thousandfold, so that I could take at one dose milliards of bacilli, very many more than one could possibly introduce by unwashed hands. Since Koch states that comma bacilli are destroyed by the acid of the gastric juice I was careful to take them on an empty stomach."[45]

To ensure stomach acid would not kill the bacteria in his "cocktail," Pettenkofer also included a bicarbonate of soda.

In the description of his experiment, von Pettenkofer also included a description of the patient: himself. He was then 74 years of age, suffered from glycosuria (sugar in the urine, perhaps a sign of diabetes) and used false teeth only for speaking, not "mastication." What if his belief was wrong, and the comma bacillus was the agent of cholera? In that event Pettenkofer would "die in the cause of science, like a soldier on the field of honour."

Pettenkofer was fortunate. Other than some diarrhea and intestinal discomfort for several days, Pettenkofer's health was seemingly unaffected. Perhaps any remaining stomach acid served to neutralize the bacteria he swallowed. Or perhaps his many years of study of cholera had rendered him immune. Even during the widespread outbreaks of cholera, not everyone exposed developed the disease. Regardless, until his death Pettenkofer remained convinced that he was right. Suffering from the growing infirmities of age coupled with melancholy, von Pettenkofer committed suicide nine years later.[46]

Others, but particularly the French and English, also remained skeptical of Koch's conclusions, even to the extent of carrying out similar self-experiments with material from rice-water stools. The British, one might argue, had much more at stake in the argument. While the French might dispute the discovery in the context of nationalism, the British were in the unenviable position of being accused of being the purveyors of the disease, first from India to Egypt, and ultimately to Europe and England itself. And as we have seen earlier in the story, it was via England, Ireland and ultimately Canada that the disease made its way through Buffalo and into Detroit. Sir William Hunter, the man who had been in charge of the British Commission which preceded that of Koch, vehe-

12. Isolation and Identification of the Cholera Bacillus

mently denied any role for a microbe, and by extension, England, asserting "his unqualified opinion that the disease was non-contagious, non-specific, and endemic in Egypt."[47] Other speakers echoed Hunter's statements. Did ships convey cholera from India? The answer was "decidedly in the negative."[48]

Noteworthy among Koch's reports is the absence of any reference to the Italian physician Filippo Pacini, who had reported the presence of the same bacillus decades prior to Koch. There is of course no evidence Koch was even aware of the earlier work, and his lack of recognition was not due to any form of malevolence. The Italians, however, were aware of the oversight: "Koch ... has dressed himself in borrowed plumes; when he 'no more, no less,' affirms that he has discovered the bacillus of cholera, discovered thirty years before by Pacini."[49]

By the time of the 9th International Sanitary Conference, held in Paris in February 1894, the issue had largely been settled, with the acknowledgement among most scientists that Koch was correct. There remained some dissenters, echoing the Pettenkofer school of thought. But even in the absence of a reliable test animal, the presence of the cholera bacillus in the excreta of victims and in the water supplies they used, became too difficult to explain in any context other than as the etiological agent of the disease. The greater issue during the 1894 conference became the question of how best to contain the spread of cholera, particularly in the Middle East. Significant emphasis was placed on the *hajj*, the Mecca pilgrimage. Between 1871 and 1893 there had been eight major cholera outbreaks along the route between Mecca and the Red Sea. By the end of the conference, despite differences with those who would never accept Koch's theory, it was acknowledged that proper sanitation, including the provision of fresh water, was helpful in limiting the spread of disease. While still premature, Koch ended the conference with a statement that the "ten year struggle over the nature of cholera was at an end."[50] The statement was overly optimistic; it was, after all, only two years after Pettenkofer and others had tested the bacillus on themselves, with minimal effect. But cholera aside, as the Golden Age of Microbiology moved to a close, disease after disease had been identified with a specific microbe, many by Koch himself and by his colleagues.

Koch's discovery of the cholera bacillus took place some 52 years after the first outbreak in Detroit. During the ten years that followed the 1892 conference there was a growing acceptance of the role played by the comma-bacillus, even among American scientists. The various theories as to the cause of cholera, many expressed earlier in this book, and the treatments that at their best at least did not kill the patient, disappeared into medical history.

13

Aftermath

By the beginning of the twentieth century nearly all the major questions about cholera had been addressed. The etiological agent had been isolated and identified, its method of transmission was understood, and the means of preventing or controlling an outbreak — proper sanitation and sewage disposal — was known as well. The last significant outbreak during this era in the United States occurred in 1911, a consequence of the sixth worldwide pandemic. During that summer cholera was widespread in Italy. In July 1911 two ships that had docked in the ports of Naples, Genoa and Palermo, the *Abruzzi* and the *Moltke*, carried passengers who had been infected. After arriving in New York, the sick passengers were removed and placed in isolation on Swinburne Island, an artificial island in New York harbor created by the addition of landfill several decades earlier. A second such site, Hoffmann Island, was likewise used for the quarantine of passengers thought to carry contagious diseases.

Eleven persons died during the outbreak, including one person who was employed at the hospital on Swinburne Island. A total of 500 passengers were screened for the cholera bacillus, with five discovered as healthy carriers. As an additional precaution to prevent such occurrences in the future, it was decided that any time a passenger on a ship from Genoa traveling to New York died while the ship was at sea, prior to the burial in the ocean, an intestinal culture would be prepared in order to determine the possible presence of cholera on the ship.[1] The 1911 outbreak in Naples was also unusual for another reason. It is perhaps the only such outbreak of cholera that was subject to governmental suppression of press coverage of an epidemic. The previous outbreak in Italy, during the 1884 pandemic, had resulted in extensive disruption to Italian society, and the Italian government appears to have made the decision in 1911 that it could avoid the same outcome by censoring any news about the current outbreak. The United States, which was happy to accept immigrants who might provide cheap labor, was alleged to have participated in the cover-up.[2] Whether this was true or not, the arrival of significant numbers of immigrants from southern Europe, including Italy, seemed to have had minimal impact on any appearance of cholera in New York that summer.

The 1911 outbreak was confined to New York, and represented the last significant incidence of cholera in the United States at a single site. Though cholera continued to rage in large portions of the world throughout the twentieth century, and still does even in the present day, the disease is largely controlled in Europe and North America. Between 1965 and 1991, the Centers for Disease Control and Prevention reported an average incidence of five cases each year in the United States. Between 1992 and 1994, as a result of the resurgence of the disease in Latin America, the average incidence rose to approximately 53 cases each year, dropping back to an average of 10 cases annually as the outbreaks in Latin America came under control. During the first decade of the twenty-first century, the annual incidence dropped even further. Nearly all the cases during this period were the result of travel to areas of the world such as Latin America in which cholera had broken out.[3] Despite a cholera scare in Detroit in 1997, that city, and Michigan in general, have been spared.[4]

The obvious means to prevent or control future outbreaks of gastrointestinal disease, not only cholera but other food or waterborne bacterial diseases as well, is the establishment of proper sanitation procedures. But scientists also understand a great deal more today about the cholera bacillus itself, including the role and molecular biology of the cholera toxin it produces. The first types of several increasingly effective vaccines against the illness were developed during the 1880s and 1890s by contemporaries Jaime Ferran y Clua and Waldemar Haffkine. Subsequent vaccines have proven safer and more effective. The toxin itself was isolated in the 1950s, and its mechanism of action elucidated during the following decades; indeed, the molecule has been proven a prototype of that class of bacterial toxins.

Since the pathology of cholera is a direct result of severe dehydration, even long before the discovery of an actual toxin, rehydration therapy, particularly fluids that replaced lost electrolytes, was shown to be

13. Aftermath

a rapid and effective means of preventing death. The form of rehydration today is determined by the extent of fluid loss and consequent clinical symptoms: none, moderate and severe.[5] If dehydration is mild, oral rehydration is sufficient; for more severe cases, intravenous therapy may be necessary. If fluids are provided in a timely manner, recovery is usually the outcome. In the absence of proper therapy, the mortality rate is still above 50 percent. This remains a particular challenge in remote or poverty-stricken areas around the world. According to figures from the World Health Organization, in 2009 some 222,000 cases were reported in 45 countries, primarily in Africa; nearly 5,000 deaths resulted. And while any deaths represent a failure in medical care, the relatively low mortality is the result of improved means of modern therapy.

Development of First Cholera Vaccine

The identification of the etiological agent meant that, in theory, it could be grown in the laboratory, inactivated, and prepared in vaccine form as a means to immunize potential victims of the disease. Certainly by the time the etiological agent of cholera was identified during the 1880s, there was precedence for vaccine production. The first vaccine was developed, or more accurately discovered, by English physician Edward Jenner, who in the 1790s observed that persons infected with the cowpox agent — the concept of a virus as a biological entity was over 100 years in the future — became immunized against smallpox. The first actual vaccines produced through manipulations of an etiological agent were the results of Louis Pasteur's work with both anthrax and rabies, several years before Koch's discovery of the cholera bacillus.

The first attempt to produce a cholera vaccine is arguably credited to Spanish physician Jaime Ferran y Clua, who during the cholera outbreak in Spain in 1884 observed that guinea pigs that survived injections of the cholera bacillus became immune to further exposure. After testing the "vaccine" on himself for determination of safety, he arranged for the manufacture of sufficient vaccine to immunize over 50,000 persons. A contemporary scientific article criticized his methods:

There seems to be little reason to suppose that the element of the body which seems to constitute the proper food of the comma bacillus can be, at least permanently, removed; for one attack of cholera affords no immunity against a second. In justice to Dr. Ferran, however, it should be said that he only claims that his system affords temporary protection. The means by which this protection is said to be secured are as follows: *by methods only known by the discoverer* [italics added], the comma bacillus is so cultivated that its spores are produced. [Note: *Vibrio* is not a spore former; Ferran was mistaken on this account.] From these spores, which are capable of enduring conditions that would prove fatal to the bacilli themselves, mulberry-like masses form, and from these masses, in turn, give birth to a generation of true bacteria. By introducing into the circulation a small quantity of liquid containing these spores, mulberry-like masses, bacilli, etc. it is said that those elements on which the comma bacillus feeds can be removed from the blood without much constitutional disturbance, thus securing an immunity against an attack of cholera until these elements can be renewed.[6]

But, to say nothing of the suspicious secrecy with which all this process is surrounded, it seems certain from the reports of those who have sought to investigate or repeat Dr. Ferran's experiments, that he is entirely ignorant, or at least careless, of the nice technical details necessary to success in the study of bacteria, and that his so-called spores are sterile and disorganized products, and therefore incapable of exerting any salutary effect as an anti-cholera inoculation.... Almost all that is known about these results is what he has chosen to tell ... for the simple reason that he has not yet secured a suitable pecuniary reward.[7]

Ferran's published results were a prime example of how not to carry out an epidemiological study. His procedure consisted of the inoculation of a small quantity of fluid — the source of the inoculum was unclear — into the arms of individuals who paid between 20 and 50 francs for the privilege of serving as a subject in Ferran's study. The number of subjects was known only by Dr. Ferran. Nor did he publish or compare the incidence of disease or death among these subjects against a control group who were not inoculated.

The responses by witnesses to Ferran's work were decidedly mixed. Some confirmed the statistics, which showed a measure of protection against the disease. Others reported significant side effects such as ulceration and pyemia (infection). Unfortunately in the rush to prepare the vaccine in the face of the impending epidemic, neither the quality nor safety was sufficiently determined by Ferran, and numerous deaths occurred even among those receiving the vaccine. A French commission, later established to evaluate Ferran's results, found them useless.[8]

Waldemar Haffkine (1860–1930) was born in Odessa, Russia, and trained as a bacteriologist with Elie Metchnikoff, later a Nobel laureate for his own studies of immunity. Haffkine's association with what was considered a radical Jewish defense group during the period in which the Russian Tsar was assassinated resulted in his leaving his Russian homeland; he eventually found a position at the Pasteur Institute in Paris, rejoining Metchnikoff, who had established a laboratory there. It was at the institute that he began his work in 1890 on development of an anticholera vaccine. Unlike the situation with Ferran, Haffkine readily described his procedures and his experimental results on animals to others in his profession. The challenge of finding an experimental animal was solved when he found that guinea pigs and rabbits could be infected with human strains of the bacillus; his experiments were subsequently modified in that Haffkine settled on a model in which he injected guinea pigs intraperitoneally (IP) to induce a disease similar to that in humans. Haffkine found that he could attenuate the microbe by treatment of cultures with either chloroform or exposure to heat. Prior exposure of guinea pigs with the attenuated forms IP was found to protect the animals against exposure to virulent strains. Haffkine further determined that subcutaneous injections could also protect the animals against virulent strains.

In July 1892 Haffkine tested his attenuated vaccine on himself, finding no significant ill effects. After further testing of the vaccine that summer and fall on some 50 volunteers, he again observed no significant side effects, and concluded the vaccine was safe. It remained only to test whether it was also effective in protecting an individual against natural exposure to the bacillus during an epidemic. It was also that fall that Haffkine had an opportunity to test the efficacy of the vaccine for himself. Mouth pipetting as a means to transfer cultures was routine for the time, even practiced by this author as a student in microbiology courses as late as the 1960s. That September Haffkine accidentally swallowed a sample of virulent bacilli. "While I was transferring with a pipette the peritoneal exudate.... I felt in my mouth the feeble, viscous, slightly salty taste of the exudate. After an instant of reflection I hurried to swallow my saliva mixed with the exudate, which is extremely rich in microbes....

Let's see if I survive the drop I just swallowed."⁹ Haffkine suffered no ill effects, concluding the vaccine was indeed efficacious.

The vaccine developed by Haffkine remained in widespread use into the 1970s. However, studies of the vaccine's efficacy found it was only 50 percent effective in conferring immunity, and even that was a relatively short-term effect. Nor did it seem to eliminate carriers. The Haffkine vaccine was useful in temporarily immunizing health-care workers in epidemic areas, but it proved to be no permanent solution to the immunization problem.

Beginning in the 1970s as the immunology of cholera was better understood, it was determined the most effective immune response was that of secretory antibody, known as IgA, produced by the intestinal mucosa. Rather than using parenteral vaccination as was practiced with the Haffkine vaccine, physicians found that vaccine administered orally was safer, more convenient, and more importantly, more effective. Two major categories of oral vaccines currently exist: killed whole-cell vaccines, with or without the inactive toxin, and genetically attenuated live vaccines that are currently (as of 2012) in the testing stage.[10] The killed whole-cell vaccines have proven effective in moderating cholera outbreaks when used properly and in a timely fashion, though long-term immunity remains unclear.

The Role of Cholera Toxin in the Pathology of the Disease

Following his isolation and description of the cholera bacillus in 1884, Robert Koch suggested the pathology of the disease may actually result from the presence of a poison, a toxin. Koch further suggested the severe diarrhea was the result of the multi-organ failure, particularly of the cardiovascular system, that resulted during the latter stages of the illness, leading to the death of the victim. Certainly there was precedent at the time for this belief — within five years of Koch's isolation of the cholera bacillus both diphtheria and tetanus were demonstrated to be the result of a systemic toxin.

In reality, Koch's explanation, later recalled as "Koch's blunder,"[11] was backward; it was the severe dehydration that ultimately resulted in

13. Aftermath

organ failure. Nevertheless, Koch's standing in the medical community at the time meant that in experimental attempts to reproduce the disease in experimental animals, scientists repeatedly injected the animals with toxin through routes other than the alimentary canal.[12] Such experiments provided little information about the disease, but did waste time and resources in its study. Since a parenterically administered culture extract could not induce fluid loss, a different explanation for the role of the bacillus developed; the pathology was due to an endotoxin, a mucinase in the vernacular of the 1950s, which constituted a portion of the structure of the bacillus. As notable a scientist as Harold Florey, awarded the 1945 Nobel Prize in Physiology or Medicine for his work with penicillin, described the effects of the toxin in such a manner: "The cholera problem is quite simple — the cholera mucinase stripped the protective layer of mucin from the intestinal epithelium, so cholera should be looked at as a kind of internal third degree burn, and no wonder that all that fluid poured into the gut."[13] The function of the toxin was finally described in 1959, when Indian scientist Sambhu Nath De applied the technique of ileal loop ligation in demonstrating the mechanism underlying the severe diarrhea characteristic of the disease. The technique, no longer used in demonstrating a mechanism of fluid loss, involved tying off a section of rabbit ileum and injecting a small volume of fluid into the site. De applied the technique in demonstrating that cell-free extracts of *Vibrio cholerae* contained the toxin, which itself induced the fluid loss typical of the disease.[14]

The molecular action of the toxin was determined a decade later. The structure of the toxin molecule is that of a protein consisting of six subunits, five of which are identical and bind the toxin to the surface of the intestinal tissue (B subunits); the sixth subunit is the active portion (A subunit), which is transported into the cell. The activity of the A subunit is twofold: it inhibits sodium uptake into the cell while increasing the secretion of chloride. The effect is a massive and rapid loss of fluid — the severe diarrhea.[15] Other features of the bacillus contribute to the pathology of the disease, but the toxin is the primary concern.

In the nearly 200 years since cholera evolved from a localized epidemic in portions of India to being associated with worldwide pandemics, nearly everything has been learned about the disease. The key to control of cholera, as it has always been, is to supply clean and fresh water, free of such contamination. But despite the belief that cholera is only a disease of poverty, it retains the potential to still infect those who deal with patients, or who may be exposed to food or water contaminated by carriers of the disease. As we have seen with the outbreaks in Latin America and Haiti, localized disasters or the endemic presence of the disease in impoverished countries means it is only a short plane trip away from anywhere else.

Chapter Notes

Introduction

1. E. Steinberg, D. Greene, C. Bopp, D. Cameron, J. Wells, and E. Mintz, "Cholera in the United States, 1995–2000: Trends at the end of the twentieth century," *Journal of Infectious Diseases* 184 (2001): 799–802.
2. http://www.cdc.gov/haiticholera/haiti_cholera.htm.
3. http://www.paho.org/english/sha/epibul_95–98/be971cho.htm.
4. *Boston Medical and Surgical Journal* 165, no. 1 (July 6, 1911): 31.
5. Wolfgang Locher, "Max von Pettenkofer — life stations of a genius on the 100th anniversary of his death (February 9, 1901)," *International Journal of Hygiene and Environmental Health* 203 (2001): 379–391.

Chapter 1

1. R. Fahraeus, "The suspension stability of blood," *Acta Medica Scandanavica* 55 (1921): 1–228, quoted in Gerald Hart, "Descriptions of blood and blood disorders before the advent of laboratory studies," *British Journal of Haematology* 115 (2001): 719–728.
2. Dhiman Barua and William B. Greenough III, eds., *Cholera* (New York, NY: Plenum, 1992), p. 1, quoting French lexicologist Paul-Maximillien-Émile Littré (1872). It should be noted Littré had studied medicine and even translated the works of Hippocrates, but was not himself a physician.
3. Kaviraj Sengupta, *The Ayurvedic System of Medicine* vol. 2 (New Delhi, India: Logos, 1994). The book was originally published in 1919, and the disagreement on the interpretation of *visuchika* is based upon his belief that "cholera is a disease which did not exist in ancient times," leaving the interpretation of "ancient" undefined.
4. Quoted in Barua and Greenough, *Cholera*, p. 3.
5. Francis Adams, trans., *The Genuine Works of Hippocrates,* vol. 1 (London: Adlard, 1849), p. 329.
6. Carlos Seas and Eduardo Gotuzzo, "The cholera epidemic in Peru and Latin America in 1991," in *Global Issues in Water, Sanitation and Health: Workshop Summary*, ed. (Washington, DC: National Academies, 2009). Also quoted by Barua and Greenough, p. 3.
7. Francis Adams, trans., *Of the Epidemics,* retrieved from http://classics.mit.edu//Hippocrates/epidemics.html.
8. Barua and Greenough, *Cholera*, p. 6.
9. S. Selwyn, "Cholera old and new," *Proceedings of the Royal Society of Medicine* 70 (1977): 301–302.
10. Steven Johnson, *The Ghost Map* (New York: Penguin, 2006), p. 33.
11. Valentine Blacker, *Memoir of the Operations of the British Army in India During the Mahratta War of 1817–1819* (London: Black, 1821), pp. 95–96.
12. "Cholera," http://www.globalsecurity.org/wmd/intro/bio_cholera.htm.
13. Christiane Bird, *The Sultan's Shadow: One Families Rule at the Crossroads of East and West* (New York: Random House, 2010), pp. 82–83.
14. Johnson, *Ghost Map*, p. 33.
15. In what became known as the November Uprising and Cadet Revolution, Polish troops, cadets and civilians began a rebellion in November 1830 against their Russian occupiers; the nation of Poland had undergone its final partition in 1795 and ceased to exist until 1918. Despite the disparity in numbers and training, the nascent

Polish army held out for most of 1831. Many of its troops entered Prussia and Austria following defeat.

16. Barua and Greenough, p. 9.

17. Cited in Joseph Barnes, et al., *The Cholera Epidemic of 1873* (Washington, DC: Government Printing Office, 1875), p. 555.

18. Charles Rosenberg, *The Cholera Years: The United States in 1832, 1849 and 1866* (Chicago: University of Chicago Press, 1987), p. 16.

19. John Woodworth, M.D., *Cholera Epidemic of 1873 in the United States* (Washington, DC: Government Printing Office, 1875), p. 558.

20. Retrieved from http://www.ph.ucla.edu/epi/snow/pandemic1826-37.html.

21. Retrieved from http://www.uppercanadahistory.ca/tt/tt1.html.

22. Goeffrey Bilson, "The first epidemic of Asiatic Cholera in Lower Canada," *Medical History* 21 (1977): 411–433.

23. Ibid., p. 416.

24. Marian Patterson, "The cholera epidemic of 1832 in York, Upper Canada," retrieved from http://www.ncbi.nlm.nih.gov/pmc/articles/PMC233409/pdf/mlab00208-1001.pdf.

25. Actually the Province of Lower Canada, formerly New France, as created in the Constitutional Act of 1791. The province of Upper Canada is largely present-day Ontario. "Upper" and "lower" refer to the direction of the St. Lawrence River. The provinces were joined in 1867.

26. Patterson, "Cholera epidemic," p. 170.

27. Bilson, "First epidemic," p. 418. From reports it is unclear where Vasseur died. Since his death is reported in church records in Quebec City, it would appear he was not on the ship.

28. Ibid., p. 419.

29. Walter Sendzik, "The 1832 Montreal cholera epidemic: A study in state formation," retrieved from http://www.collectionscanada.gc.ca/obj/s4/f2/dsk2/ftp01/MQ37236.pdf.

30. *La Minerve,* June 14, 1832, cited in "retrieved from http://www.cbc.ca/history/EPISCONTENTSE1EP7CH1PA5LE.html.

31. *Democratic Free Press,* July 12, 1832, p. 2.

32. Bilson, "First epidemic," p. 420.

33. *La Minerve.*

34. Bilson, "First epidemic," p. 420.

35. Joseph Barnes, et al., *The Cholera Epidemic in the United States in 1873* (Washington, DC: Government Printing Office, 1875), p. 566.

Chapter 2

1. Barnes, *Cholera Epidemic,* p. 566. Barnes' source appears to have been Lewis Beck, "Report on cholera," *Transactions of the Medical Society of the State of New York,* August 1832, 348–372.

2. Beck, "Report on cholera," 348–372.

3. Ibid.

4. Ashleigh Tuite, Christina Chan, and David Fisman, "Cholera, canals, and contagion: Rediscovering Dr. Beck's report," *Journal of Public Health Policy* 32 (2011): 320–333.

5. Ibid., p. 567. Alexander Francis Vache, M.D. (1800–1857), was practicing in New York at this time. See also Charles Rosenberg, *The Cholera Years* (Chicago: University of Chicago Press, 1962), p. 25n.

6. The original Erie Canal stretched some 363 miles, connecting Albany, New York, on the Hudson River, with Buffalo on Lake Erie. Construction of the canal represented one of the most challenging engineering feats in nineteenth century America. Construction began in July 1817 and was completed by October 1825. In addition to the cost of building the canal, the geography of upper New York State as well as ever-present disease associated with mosquitoes and marshland presented additional challenges. An excellent resource for the general reader interested in the history of the canal's construction can be found in Gerard Koeppel, *Bond of Union: Building the Erie Canal and the American Empire* (Cambridge, MA: Da Capo, 2009). The purpose of the canal was to connect the Great Lakes and interior states and territories with the Atlantic Ocean, as well as more rapid transportation to the growing American interior. Directly and indirectly, commerce from the interior played a significant role in the final boundaries established during the nineteenth century for

Notes — Chapter 2

those states that bordered or required greater access to the Great Lakes: New York, Pennsylvania, Ohio, Michigan, Indiana, Wisconsin and Minnesota (Mark Stein, *How the States Got Their Shapes* [New York, NY: HarperCollins, 2008], and *How the States Got Their Shapes Too: The People Behind the Borderlines* [Washington, DC: Smithsonian, 2011]).

7. Matthew Algeo, *The President Is a Sick Man* (Chicago, IL: Chicago Review, 2011), p. 21.

8. Lewis Allen, "First appearance in 1832 of the cholera in Buffalo," *Publications of the Buffalo Historical Society*, vol. 4 (Buffalo, NY: Peter Paul, 1896), pp. 245–256.

9. Black Rock was a village northwest of Buffalo in 1832. It was later incorporated into the city of Buffalo.

10. Allen, "First appearance."

11. Samuel Manning Welch, *Home History: Recollections of Buffalo During the Decade from 1830 to 1840, or Fifty Years Since* (Buffalo: Peter Paul & Bro, 1890), p. 265.

12. Ibid., p. 266.

13. Ibid.

14. Ibid., p. 267.

15. Stephen Powell, "The Cholera epidemic of 1832," *The Buffalonian*, retrieved from http://www.buffalonian.com/history/articles/1801–50/cholera32.html. It was a common belief of the time that cholera mainly attacked the outcasts of society, especially those perceived as drunkards—the pejorative description of the Irish — or shiftless. To prevent exposure doctors advised citizens to avoid whiskey and to keep windows closed at night in order to prevent "miasmas" or bad air from carrying the infection.

16. Barnes, *Cholera Epidemic*, p. 568.

17. Allen, "First Appearance."

18. Ibid.

19. Ibid.

20. Frank Stevens, *The Black Hawk War* (Chicago: Frank E. Stevens, 1903), p. 242; Order No. 51, Adjutant General's Office, Washington, DC, June 16, 1832.

21. Ellen Whitney, ed., *The Black Hawk War 1831–1832*, vol. 2, *Letters and Papers, Part 1* (Springfield, IL: Illinois State Historical Library, 1973), pp. 599–601. The specific orders read, "The commanding officer of Fort Monroe will detach five companies from the Artillery School of Practice prepared and equipped for active service as Infantry, with orders to proceed forthwith to Fort Dearborn, Chicago, via New York and the Lakes. The battalion will be commanded by Brevet Lieutenant-Colonel Crane of the 4th Regiment of Artillery.... Brevet Major Payne, with his company, will proceed forthwith to Fort Columbus [now Governor's island, New York City], and on being there joined by companies ... of the 4th Artillery ... will resume the line of march for Chicago. The Garrisons of Forts Niagara [junction of Niagara River and Lake Ontario] and Gratiot [north of Detroit] to be conducted by their respective commandants, Lieutenant-Colonel [Alexander] Cummings and Brevet Major [Alexander] Thompson, of the 2nd Regiment of Infantry, will forthwith proceed to Chicago; and one company of the 5th Regiment from each of the Garrisons of Forts Brady [Sault St. Marie River in northern Michigan] and Mackinac [Mackinac Island, northern Michigan], will be detached, and be ordered ... to the same point of Rendezvous." Thompson was killed in 1837 during the Seminole Wars.

"Surgeon [Josiah] Everett is assigned to duty with the battalion of Artillery ordered from Fort Monroe; and Assistant Surgeon [Edward] Macomb, to the detachment from Fort McHenry [Baltimore], and the harbor of New York."

"Brevet Major General [Winfield] Scott is charged with the execution of this order, and the prompt movement of the several detachments herein ordered from the sea board and upper lakes. General Scott will repair to Chicago, assume command of the forces, and direct the operations against the hostile Indians. By order: R. [Roger] Jones Adjutant General."

22. Jean Loehde, retrieved fromhttp://files.usgwarchives.net/mi/downward/multiple/ships/c40002.txt. Scott originally planned to hire three steamboats. Major Alexander Thompson at Fort Gratiot was to engage a fourth boat, pick up additional troops from Fort Brady in northern Michigan, and from there travel to Chicago via Lake Michigan.

23. Retrieved from http://ech.cwru.edu/ech-cgi/article.pl?id=CEO1.

24. *Medical Statistics United States Army*, 1840, p. 91, cited in Edmund Charles Wendt, ed., *A Treatise on Asiatic Cholera* (New York, NY: William Wood, 1885), p. 72.

25. Twiggs was born in Georgia in 1790. He served honorably in the War of 1812, in the Seminole wars, in the Black Hawk War and later in the war with Mexico, despite becoming embroiled in an issue over rank. Twiggs attained a level of infamy during the months preceding the Civil War when, in February 1861, he surrendered military posts in Texas to Colonel Ben McCulloch and the future Confederate Army there. President James Buchanan dismissed Twiggs from the army "for treachery to the flag of his country" retrieved from http://www.jstor.org/pss/30235761).

26. Payne was commander at Fort McHenry at Baltimore. The fort of course is well known in American history for its role in the War of 1812 while flying the "Star-Spangled Banner."

27. Barnes, *Cholera Epidemic*, p. 569. While one hesitates to invoke the superstition of a boat being cursed, the history of the *Henry Clay* would appear to fit within that category. Prior to the appearance of cholera on board during the events of July 1832, the boat had already been subject to its fair share of wrecks. The *Henry Clay*'s story culminated on July 28, 1852, when, as it traveled from Albany to New York, a fire broke out that quickly engulfed the entire boat. Panic ensued before the captain could run the boat aground, and sixty passengers, including the sister of writer Nathaniel Hawthorne, died.

28. Eustis was the first commander of Fortress Monroe, appointed in 1830. He later commanded the school for artillery practice at that fort. As was the case with many of General Scott's associates, Crane had distinguished himself in the fighting during the War of 1812, being instrumental in the capture of forts York and George in Canada. During the period of the Black Hawk War, Crane was permanent commander of Fort Columbus in New York harbor. Worth was an aide and close friend of Scott's, naming his son Winfield Scott Worth after the general. He was partially lame much of his life, the result of a severe wound acquired during the War of 1812. Worth later distinguished himself during both the Second Seminole War in Florida during the 1830s and the Mexican War. Worth and Scott had serious disagreements over tactics in the latter war, an argument so serious that Worth even changed the name of his son to William.

29. Beck, "Report on cholera," p. 361.

30. Ibid., p. 362.

31. Ibid.

32. Silas Farmer, *History of Detroit and Wayne County*, 3rd ed. (Detroit: Silas Farmer, 1890). The first post road in the territory ran between Detroit and Cincinnati, and had been established in 1801.

33. William Jenks, "Fort Gratiot and its builder Gen. Charles Gratiot," *Michigan History Magazine* 4 (1920): 141–155.

Chapter 3

1. W. O'Shaughnessy, "Proposal of a new method of treating the blue epidemic cholera by the injection of highly-oxygenises salts into the venous system," *The Lancet* 17 (December 3, 1831): 366–371. A summary of Latta's work is provided in N. MacGillivray, "Dr Latta of Leith: Pioneer in the Treatment of Cholera by Intravenous Saline Infusion," *Journal of the Royal College of Physicians of Edinburgh* 36 (2006): 80–85.

2. The complete list of names of cadets who accompanied Scott is as follows: George Ward, 2nd Artillery; Edward Deas, 4th Artillery; Ward Burnett, 2nd Artillery; Richard Fain, 1st Artillery; Henderson Yoakum, 3rd Artillery; Henry Sill, 1st Artillery; Joseph Vance, 2nd Artillery; George Watson, 1st Artillery; Franklin McDuffee, 4th Artillery (died July 15 at Fort Dearborn in present-day Chicago); Lewis Howell, 7th Artillery; William Wall, 3rd Artillery; John Macomb, 4th Artillery; Tench Tilghman, 4th Artillery; Lorenzo Sitgreaves, 1st Artillery; George Crittenden, 4th Infantry; Jacob Brown, 2nd Infantry; Randolph Marcy, 5th Infantry; James Hardin, 4th Infantry; Roger Dix, 7th Infantry; James Bomford, 2nd Infantry; Richard Gatlin, 7th Infantry; George Griffin, 6th Infantry; William Kello, 3rd Infantry; Henry Swart-

wout, 3rd Infantry; Gaines Kingsbury, Mtd. Rangers; Humphrey Marshall, Mtd. Rangers; James Bowman, Mtd. Rangers; Ashburn Ury, Mtd. Rangers; and Albert Edwards, Mtd. Rangers. A few of these cadets would later be noted for their service in the Mexican War and the Civil War.

John Wentworth, *Early Chicago, Fort Dearborn: An Address Delivered at the Unveiling of the Memorial, May 21st, 1881* (Chicago: Fergus, 1881), Appendix J.

3. Whitney, *Black Hawk War*, p. 736. The actual title for the section was "Economy of an army on campaign," as revised in 1821 under Secretary of War John C. Calhoun. The sections addressed topics such as organization of the troops, necessities for the officers, movement of provisions and baggage, disposition during battle and methods for handling of prisoners. *General Regulations for the Army; or Military Institutes* (Philadelphia: M. Carey, 1821). The manual underwent some revision in 1825, and was presumably that under which Scott issued his orders.

4. The island is located in the Detroit River just east of Detroit. The site has undergone a number of name changes since it was originally occupied by the Chippewa and Ottawa, Native American tribes who named it Wa-na-be-zee (Swan Island). It acquired the name Hog Island from the French (*Ile au Cochons*), since the first French settlers housed pigs and chickens on site to avoid predators on the mainland. In 1845 Barnabus Campau, who had purchased the site several decades earlier, renamed the island Belle Isle (Beautiful Island), the name by which it is known today. It became the first public park in Detroit in 1884 and for many years has been the site of a large picnic area and a zoo.

5. Woodworth, *Cholera Epidemic of 1873*, pp. 570–571.

6. Ibid.

7. In addition to Clay and Everett, others who died from cholera during the week included 2nd Lieutenant Gustavus Brown, Class of 1829, United States Military Academy, 3rd Artillery on July 12th at Fort Dearborn; and Brevet 2nd Lieutenant Franklin McDuffie, 4th Artillery, on July 15 (*American Railroad Journal*, July 1832–January 1833, p. 713).

8. Sergeant Christain Heyl (sic) was born in New York ca. 1799. He had enlisted at Fort Monroe on February 9, 1832. Little is known about Heyl beyond the description of his death. He was tall for the time — 6'2" — and given his rank had likely served earlier (ancestry.com).

9. Whitney, *Black Hawk War*, p. 781.

10. Augustus Walker, "Early days on the lake," *Publications of the Buffalo Historical Society* 5: 287–315.

11. Arthur Smith, *Old Fuss and Feathers: The Life and Exploits of Lt.-General Winfield Scott* (New York: Greystone, 1937), p. 176.

12. Milo Quaife, *Chicago and the Old Northwest: 1673–1835* (Chicago: University of Chicago Press, 2009), p. 331; Wentworth, *Early Chicago*, p. 37.

13. Edmund Charles Wendt, ed., *A Treatise on Asiatic Cholera*, (New York, NY: William Wood, 1885), p. 72.

Chapter 4

1. Almon Parkins, *The Historical Geography of Detroit* (Chicago: The University of Chicago, 1918), p. 144–182.

2. Silas Farmer, *History of Detroit and Wayne County and Early Michigan: A Chronological Cyclopedia of the Past and Present* (Detroit: Silas Farmer, 1890), pp. 60–61.

3. http://wayne.migenweb.net/board index.htm.

4. Michael Daisy, ed., *Detroit Water and Sewerage Department: The First 300 Years*, retrieved from http://www.dwsd.org/downloads_n/about_dwsd/history/complete_history.pdf.

5. Ibid.

6. Ibid.

7. Ibid.

8. Ibid. Holes were drilled into the wood to allow fire crews to connect their hoses. When finished, the holes were "plugged." Thus the name fire plug was coined.

9. Ibid., p. 60.

10. Arthur Woodford, *This is Detroit: 1701–2001* (Detroit, MI: Wayne State University Press, 2001), p. 2.

11. George Newman Fuller, *Economic and Social Beginnings of Michigan* (Lansing,

Notes—Chapter 5

MI: Wynkoop, Hallenbeck Crawford, 1916), p. 134.

12. *Journal of the Proceedings of the Common Council of the City of Det*roit, 1824–1843, pp. 50–52, cited in Fuller, *Economic and Social Beginnings,* p. 136.

13. Joseph Molner and Vlado Getting, "Medical Care Functions of the Detroit Health Department," *American Journal of Public Health* 45 (July 1955): 855–861.

14. *Journal of the Michigan State Medical Society* 12 (April 1913): 222.

15. Molner and Getting, "Medical care functions," p. 855.

16. *Democratic Free Press,* October 6, 1831, p. 2. Note also use of the term *vaccinate* in the report. The term was used in honoring Edward Jenner, the British country physician who some thirty years earlier had discovered a means to prevent smallpox through immunization with the lymph of cowpox, an infection on the udders of cattle—*vacca* in Latin. Louis Pasteur is often given credit for coining the term vaccination some fifty years later. Clearly it was in use before that.

17. Chapin (1798–1838) served as mayor from 1831–1832. He was appointed to the position of city physician during the cholera outbreaks of 1832 and 1834. During this period Chapin was also the proprietor of a drug store. He was also well known for the impressive garden he maintained. Included among his plants was what was sometimes called the "love-apple," grown for ornamental purposes only as it was considered poisonous by some. The more familiar name was "tomato."

18. Silas Farmer, *The History of Detroit and Michigan or The Metropolis Illustrated: A Chronological Cyclopedia of the Past and Present* (Detroit: Silas Farmer, 1884), p. 59.

19. *Democratic Free Press,* March 8, 1832, p. 1.

Chapter 5

1. David Herbert Donald, *Lincoln* (New York, NY: Touchstone, 1996), p. 45.

2. Retrieved from http://www.illinoisgenealogy.org/rock-island/general_gaines_reply_to_gov_reynolds.htm.

3. John Reynolds, *My Own Times: Embracing Also the History of My Life* (Chicago: Chicago Historical Society, 1855, pp. 344–45.

4. Ibid.

5. Charles Winslow Elliott, *Winfield Scott, The Soldier and the Man* (New York, NY: Macmillan, 1937), pp. 260–64.

6. Robert Braun, "Black Hawk's War, April 5—August 2, 1832: A chronology," *Old Lead Historical Society,* September 2001.

7. A monument at the site in Stillman Valley, Illinois, now listed on the National Register of Historic Places, includes a plaque inscribed, "In memory of the Illinois volunteers who fell at Stillman's Run, May 14, 1832, in an engagement with Black Hawk and his warriors." Also inscribed is, "The presence of soldier, statesman, martyr, Abraham Lincoln assisting in the burial of these honored dead has made this spot more sacred."

8. E. Buckner, "A brief history of the war with the Sac and Fox Indians in Illinois and Michigan in 1832," *Michigan Historical Collections* 12 (1887): 424–436. Also an excellent first-person account of the conflict.

9. In 1832 that portion of Wisconsin was part of Michigan Territory.

10. Henry Colin Campbell, *Wisconsin in Three Centuries, 1634–1905: Wisconsin as a Territory* (New York, NY: Publishing Society of New York, 1906), p. 200.

11. Reynolds, *My Own Times,* p. 419.

12. Irving Burton, "The cholera epidemic in Detroit 1832 and 1834," *Michigan Medicine,* October 1969, 1013–21.

13. *Democratic Free Press,* July 12, 1832, p. 2.

14. Corlaer's Hook was located on the Lower East Side of New York City, jutting into the East River across from Long Island. It was named Crown Point at the time of the revolution. The hospital was a converted workshop used to house cholera patients that summer of 1832. The area was also famous for its streetwalkers, and the term "hooker" may have originated there.

15. *New York Journal,* cited *in Democratic Free Press,* August 23, 1832, p. 3.

16. Burton, "The cholera epidemic"; *Democratic Free Press,* July 12, 1832, p. 2.

17. Joseph K. Barnes, et al., *The Cholera Epidemic of 1873 in the United States* (Washington, D.C.: Government Printing Office, 1875), p. 570.

18. Friend Palmer, *Early Days in Detroit* (Detroit, MI: Hunt and June, 1906), p. 281.
19. *Chicago Tribune*, February 8, 1861, p. 2.
20. Palmer, *Early Days*, p. 571.
21. *Democratic Free Press*, July 12, 1832, p. 2.
22. Burton, "The cholera epidemic."
23. *Democratic Free Press*, July 12, 1832, p. 2.
24. *Democratic Free Press*, August 2, 1832, p. 3.
25. Burton, "The cholera epidemic."
26. Retrieved from http://clarke.cmich.edu/resource_tab/information_and_exhibits/i_arrived_at_detroit/emily_mason.html.
27. Bill Loomis, *Detroit's Delectable Past: Two Centuries of Frog Legs, Pigeon Pie and Drugstore Whiskey* (Charleston, SC: History Press, 2012), p. 162.
28. Letter, Samuel B. Smith to Capt. Wilson, *Niles' Weekly Register* 43 (November 24, 1832): 203. Smith had been stationed at Fort Armstrong at Rock Island during the 1832 epidemic.
29. Palmer, *Early Days*, p. 281.
30. Loomis, *Detroit's Delectable Past*, p. 162.
31. C.M. Burton, "Detroit in the year 1832," *Michigan Historical Collections* 28 (1898): 163–171.
32. Retrieved from http://files.usgwarchives.net/mi/lenawee/history/petition2.txt.
33. *Democratic Free Press*, October 25, 1832, p. 1.
34. *Democratic Free Press*, September 27, 1832, p. 1.
35. *Democratic Free Press*, November 15, 1832, p. 1.
36. *History of Washtenaw County Michigan* (Chicago: Charles Chapman, 1881), p. 594.
37. Lawton Hemans, *Life and Times of Stevens Thomson Mason, the Boy Governor of Michigan* (Lansing, MI: Michigan Historical Commission, 1920), pp. 82–83.
38. *History of Washtenaw County Michigan*, pp. 594–95.
39. *Democratic Free Press*, July 19, 1832, p. 2.
40. JS Collection, LDS Church History Library.
41. Palmer, *Early Days*, p. 283.
42. H.M. Hughes, "Calomel treatment of cholera," *American Journal of the Medical Sciences* 37 no. 1 (January 1850): 258.
43. Loomis, *Detroit's Delectable Past*, p. 164. Chase was a prominent physician in Ann Arbor for many years, most noted for a number of recipe booklets he published.
44. Ibid., p. 163.
45. *Democratic Free Press*, August 2, 1832, p. 3.
46. *Democratic Free Press*, July 19, 1832, p. 2.
47. Ibid.
48. *Democratic Free Press*, July 12, 1832, p. 2. The Reverend P.W. Warriner was pastor of the church of Monroe. The Presbytery of Detroit had been organized in September 1828, and embraced the entire Michigan Territory at the time (William Boyd, *Historical Narrative* [Monroe, MI: Commercial Printing House, 1885], pp. 3–4).
49. *Democratic Free Press*, September 27, 1832, p. 3.
50. Michigan Pioneer and Historical Society, *Historical Collections*, vol. 28 (Lansing, MI: Robert Smith, 1900), p. 170.

Chapter 6

1. Hewson Peeke, "Chapter 14: The three cholera years," in *A Standard History of Erie County, Ohio* (Chicago and New York: Lewis, 1916).
2. *Democratic Free Press*, July 9, 1834, p. 2.
3. Friend Palmer, *Early Days in Detroit* (Detroit: Hunt and June, 1906), p. 282.
4. *Democratic Free Press*, August 13, 1834, p. 2.
5. Ibid.
6. Ibid.
7. *Democratic Free Press*, August 27, 1834, p. 2.
8. *Democratic Free Press*, August 20, 1834, p. 2.
9. *Medical History of Michigan, Michigan State Medical Society*, Vol. 1 (Minneapolis and St. Paul, MN: Bruce, 1903), p. 715.
10. Paul Leake, *A History of Detroit*, vol. 1 (Chicago and New York: Lewis, 1912), p. 416.

11. Peter Morris, *Baseball Fever: Early Baseball in Michigan* (Ann Arbor, MI: University of Michigan Press, 2003), pp. 23–25.
12. William Bunge, *Fitzgerald: Geography of a Revolution* (Athens, GA: University of Georgia Press, 2011), p. 10.
13. Palmer, *Early Days*, pp. 730–31.
14. David Chardavoyne, *A Hanging in Detroit: Stephen Gifford Simmons and the Last Execution Under Michigan Law* (Detroit, MI: Wayne State University Press, 2003), pp. 113–16.
15. *Democratic Free Press*, August 13, 1834, p. 3.
16. Palmer, *Early Days*, p. 283.
17. Letters of J. Dean (1854); Burton Collection, Detroit Public Library.
18. Palmer, *Early Days*, p. 285.
19. *Historical Collections, Michigan Pioneer and Historical Society*, vol. 35 (Lansing, MI: Wynkoop Hallenbeck Crawford, 1907), p. 250.
20. Clarence Burton, ed., *The City of Detroit, Michigan, 1701–1922*, vol. 5 (Detroit, MI: S.J. Clarke, 1922), p. 426.
21. *Historical Collections, Michigan Pioneer and Historical Society*, vol. 26 (Lansing, MI: Wynkoop Hallenbeck Crawford, 1907), p. 269–70.
22. *Democratic Free Press*, September 17, 1834, p. 3.
23. Ibid., p. 2.
24. Palmer, *Early Days*, p. 285.
25. Burton, *City of Detroit*, vol. 2, p. 1387.
26. *Democratic Free Press*, October 22, 1834, p. 3.
27. Allan Nevins and Milton Halsey Thomas, eds., *The Diary of George Templeton Strong*, vol. 4 (New York: Macmillan, 1952), pp. 96–97, cited in Charles Rosenberg, *The Cholera Years: The United States in 1832, 1849 and 1866* (Chicago, IL: University of Chicago Press, 1962), p. 217.

Chapter 7

1. Earl Kleinschmidt, "Prevailing diseases and hygienic conditions in early Michigan," *Pioneer Health* 25 (1941): 57–99.
2. *Detroit Free Press*, December 28, 1848, p. 2.
3. *Michigan Journal of Homeopathy* 1 (1848), p. 44, cited in Kleinschmidt, "Prevailing diseases," pp. 69–70.
4. Silas Farmer, *The History of Detroit and Michigan* (Detroit: Silas Farmer, 1884), p. 50.
5. Paul Leake, *History of Detroit*, vol. 1 (Chicago and New York: Lewis, 1912), p. 417.
6. Ibid., pp. 417–18.
7. *Democratic Free Press*, March 7, 1844, p. 2.
8. Ibid., February 21, 1844, p. 2.
9. Leake, *History of Detroit*, vol. 1, pp. 417–48.
10. *Detroit Free Press*, January 3, 1850, p. 2.
11. Lemuel Shattuck, *Report of the Sanitary Commission of Massachusetts 1850* (Boston: Dutton and Wentworth, 1850), pp. 33–34, retrieved from http://www.deltaomega.org/documents/shattuck.pdf. A portion of the quote is also cited in Michael Willrich, *Pox: An American History* (New York: Penguin, 2011), p. 257.
12. *Detroit Free Press*, August 23, 1850, p. 2. Founded in 1850, the Female Medical College was the first such degree-granting agency in the country. In 1867 it was renamed the Women's Medical College of Pennsylvania. It continues today as the Allegheny University of the Health Sciences.
13. Robert Roberts, *Sketches of the City of Detroit* (Detroit: R.F. Johnstone, 1855), pp. 39–40.
14. Patricia Rushton, "Cholera and its impact on nineteenth-century Mormon migration," *BYU Studies* 44, no. 2 (2005): 123–144, retrieved from https://byustudies.byu.edu/PDFLibrary/44.2RushtonCholera-bb78b7fe-2282-41c9-9ab0-c09b34018536.pdf.
15. John Kelly, *The Graves Are Walking: The Great Famine and the Saga of the Irish People* (New York: Henry Holt, 2012), p. 260.
16. Ibid., p. 264.
17. Bruce Haley, *The Healthy Body and Victorian Culture* (Cambridge, MA: Harvard University Press, 1978).
18. Retrieved from http://www.sciencemuseum.org.uk/hommedia.ashx?id=7498&size=Large.
19. Kelly, *Graves Are Walking*, p. 272.

Chapter 8

1. Edmund Charles Wendt, *A Treatise on Asiatic Cholera* (New York: William Wood, 1885).
2. Ibid., p. 27.
3. *Detroit Free Press*, December 18, 1848, p. 2.
4. *Detroit Free Press*, December 22, 1848, p. 2.
5. *Detroit Free Press*, January 9, 1849, p. 2.
6. *Cincinnati Commercial*, January 6, 1849, quoted in the *Detroit Free Press*, January 17, 1849, p. 2.
7. Wendt, *Treatise*, p. 28.
8. *Detroit Free Press*, January 19, 1849, p. 2.
9. Charles E. Rosenberg, *The Cholera Years: The United States in 1832, 1849, and 1866* (Chicago, IL: University of Chicago Press, 1962), p. 104.
10. Ibid., p. 106.
11. Ibid., p. 108.
12. *Detroit Free Press*, April 3, 1849, p. 2.
13. *Detroit Free Press*, May 9, 1849, p. 2.
14. *Detroit Free Press*, June 1, 1849, p. 2.
15. *Detroit Free Press*, May 22, 1849, p. 2.
16. *Detroit Free Press*, June 20, 1849, p. 2.
17. *The Eclectic Medical Journal* 1, no. 6 (June 1849): 273–75. Eclectic medicine largely eschewed the use of the more radical forms of treatments, including those that utilized mercury compounds. The preference was for the use of herbs or other "natural" forms of treatment. Byrd's advocacy of sulfur would not have been out of line with such thought.
18. Rosenberg, *Cholera Years*, p. 152.
19. *Detroit Free Press*, June 6, 1849, p. 3.
20. Clarence Monroe Burton, *Detroit in 1849*, collection of newspaper accounts, 1910, University of Michigan Library.
21. Samuel Duffield, "Emanations of sewers a secret cause of disease," *Detroit Review of Medicine and Pharmacy* 4, no. 9 (September 1869): 397–400.
22. *Detroit Free Press*, October 5, 1849, p. 2.

Chapter 9

1. Edmund Wendt, ed., *A Treatise on Asiatic Cholera* (New York: William Wood, 1885), p. 33.
2. Ibid.
3. Zina Pitcher, "The cholera of 1854, in Detroit," *Peninsular Journal of Medicine and the Collateral Sciences* 2, no. 4 (October 1854): 145–151. The Peninsular Medical Society, which published the journal, was organized in 1853. Its membership reached a peak of 115 physicians before being disbanded in 1860.
4. *Detroit Daily Free Press*, June 20, 1854, p. 2.
5. Ibid., p. 3.
6. Pitcher, "Cholera of 1854," pp. 146–47.
7. In fact there were at least eleven deaths attributed to cholera during this period in Ann Arbor, primarily of travelers from areas in which the disease was present (ibid., pp. 111–12).
8. *Detroit Daily Free Press*, May 28, 1854, p. 3.
9. Silas Farmer, *The History of Detroit and Michigan* (Detroit: Silas Farmer, 1884), pp. 69–70.
10. Pitcher, "Cholera of 1854," p. 149.
11. Ibid., pp. 147–48.
12. *Detroit Daily Free Press*, July 23, 1854, p. 3.
13. Retrieved from http://familytreemaker.genealogy.com/users/s/t/o/Mary-jo-Stoutenburg/PDFGENE6.pdf.
14. Earl Kleinschmidt, "Prevailing diseases and hygienic conditions in early Michigan," *Michigan History* 25 (1941): 72.
15. Pitcher, "Cholera of 1854," pp. 148–49.
16. Ibid., p. 150.
17. Ibid.
18. Ibid., p. 151.
19. Frederic Lente, "On the sedative action of calomel in disease," *New York Medical Journal* 11, no. 1 (March 1870): 11.
20. A.G. Lawton, "On the epidemic cholera," *The American Medical Monthly* 3 (March 1855): 174–87.
21. W.J. Anderson, "On the use of nitrosulphuric acid in cholera and diarrhea," *Association Medical Journal* 1, no. 44 (November 4, 1853): 964–965.

22. *Christian Inquirer,* September 2, 1854, p. 1.
23. Samuel Hahnemann, *Organon of Medicine* (Blaine, WA: Cooper, 1982).
24. Samuel Hahnemann, *The Lesser Writings of Samuel Hahnemann* (New York: William Radde, 1852), pp. 756–57.
25. Ibid., pp. 758–60.
26. Ibid., p. 760.
27. Ibid., p. 762.
28. Alonzo Palmer and Edmund Andrews, eds., *Peninsular Journal of Medicine and the Collateral Sciences* 2, no. 11 (May 1855): 502–07.
29. *Detroit Free Press,* July 11, 1884, p. 3.

Chapter 10

1. *Detroit Daily Free Press,* March 7, 1858, p. 1.
2. *Detroit Daily Free Press,* September 8, 1865, p. 1.
3. Earl Kleinschmidt, "Prevailing diseases and hygienic conditions in early michigan," *Michigan History* 25 (1941): 57–99.
4. *Detroit Free Press,* November 11, 1865, p. 1.
5. *Detroit Free Press,* November 14, 1865, p. 2.
6. *Detroit Free Press,* November 24, 1865, p. 1.
7. Kleinschmidt, "Prevailing diseases," p. 75.
8. Samuel Duffield, "Emanations of sewers a secret cause of disease," *Detroit Review of Medicine and Pharmacy* 4, no. 9 (September 1869): 397–400.
9. Ibid. Crookes was physicist William Crookes, president of the British Royal Society, and most noted for development of the Crookes tube for demonstrating ionizing radiation. During the 1860s he was involved in the study of cattle plague (likely rinderpest), including the attempt to use carbolic acid as a means of treating the disease.
10. Charles Rosenberg, *The Cholera Years: The United States in 1832, 1849 and 1866* (Chicago, IL: University of Chicago Press, 1962), p. 198.
11. Theo McGraw, "Aetiology of cholera," *Medical and Surgical Reporter* 14, no. 6 (February 10, 1866): 110. Translation of article by Felix von Niemeyer.
12. *Detroit Free Press,* November 8, 1865, p. 1.
13. McGraw, "Aetiology of cholera."
14. Joseph Barnes, *The Cholera Epidemic in the United States in 1873* (Washington: Government Printing Office, 1875), p. 660.
15. Ibid., p. 661.
16. *The New York Times,* April 23, 1866, p. 4.
17. Barnes, *Cholera Epidemic,* p. 662.
18. Ibid.
19. Ibid., p. 663.
20. Rosenberg, *Cholera Years,* pp. 184–85.
21. Ibid.
22. Ibid.
23. John Kelly, *The Graves Are Walking* (New York: Henry Holt, 2012), p. 267.
24. Retrieved from http://www.vny.cuny.edu/index-2.html.
25. Barnes, *Cholera Epidemic,* p. 664.
26. *Detroit Free Press,* August 3, 1866, p. 2.
27. Barnes, *Cholera Epidemic,* p. 665.
28. *Detroit Free Press,* May 31, 1866, p. 3.
29. *Detroit Free Press,* August 6, 1866, p. 2.
30. *Detroit Free Press,* April 13, 1866, p. 1.
31. Kleinschmidt, "Prevailing diseases," p. 76.
32. *Detroit Free Press,* June 26, 1866, p. 5.
33. *Detroit Free Press,* August 4, 1866, p. 5.
34. *Detroit Free Press,* August 29, 1866, p. 5.
35. *Detroit Free Press,* April 28, 1867, p. 2. While the concept of bath houses never developed beyond the planning stages in Detroit, the nearby city of Mt. Clemens, situated on the sites of mineral springs, did establish the first such bath houses in the state beginning in 1873. Mt. Clemens later acquired the name "Bath City of America."
36. A.B. Palmer, *Epidemic Cholera: Its Pathology and Treatment* (Detroit: William Graham, 1866).
37. Ibid., pp. 3–4.
38. Ibid., p. 4.
39. Ibid., p. 5.
40. Ibid.

41. *The Medical Times and Gazette* 1 (February 3, 1866), p. 133.
42. John Sharpe Chambers, *The Conquest of Cholera: America's Greatest Scourge* (New York: Macmillan, 1938), cited in R. Pollitzer, "Cholera Studies: I. History of the Disease," *Bulletin of the World Health Organization* 10 (1954): 421–61.

Chapter 11

1. Edmund Charles Wendt, *A Treatise on Asiatic Cholera* (New York: William Wood, 1885).
2. *Detroit Free Press*, April 15, 1873, p. 1.
3. *Detroit Free Press*, June 18, 1873, p. 2.
4. *Detroit Free Press*, August 6, 1876, p. 3.
5. *Detroit Free Press*, December 18, 1884, p. 7.
6. Ibid., p. 4.
7. *Detroit Free Press*, July 17, 1884, p. 8.
8. *13th Annual Report of the Secretary of the State Board of Health of the State of Michigan, for the fiscal year ending September 30, 1885* (Lansing: Thorp and Godfrey, 1886), pp. 196–97.
9. Ibid.
10. *Detroit Free Press*, July 18, 1885, p. 2.

Chapter 12

1. Steven Johnson, *The Ghost Map: The Story of London's Most Terrifying Epidemic—and How It Changed Science, Cities, and the Modern World* (New York: Riverhead, 2006); while we often visualize the "Victorian Age," the sixty-four years of Victoria's reign, as one of intense morality, the image is more in line with the views of Albert, the Prince Consort. Victoria herself was quite progressive, even modern as we think of the term (Stanley Weintraub, *Victoria: An Intimate Biography* [New York, NY: Dutton Adult/Penguin, 1987]).
2. John Snow, *On the Mode of Communication of Cholera*, 2nd ed. (London: John Churchill, 1855).
3. Ibid.
4. Ibid., p. 47.
5. "John Snow, the Broad Street pump and after," in *The Epidemiological Imagination*, ed. John Ashton (Bristol, PA: Open University Press, 1994), pp. 2–5.
6. Ibid., p. 51.
7. Ibid., p. 52.
8. J.P. Vandenbroucke, Rooda Eelkman, and H. Beukers, "Who made John Snow a hero?" *American Journal of Epidemiology* 133, no. 10 (May 15, 1991): 967–73.
9. "Why did you have the presumption to think that you could isolate an enzyme when so many of our great German chemists have failed?" (James B. Sumner, "The story of urease," *Journal of Chemical Education* 14, no. 6 [1937]: 255–59). Sumner, a Nobel laureate, described the challenge that he, an American chemist, had in convincing German chemists of the interpretation of his discovery that enzymes were proteins.
10. Bruno Atalic, "1885 cholera controversy: Klein versus Koch," *Journal of Medical Ethics; Medical Humanities* 36 (2010): 43–47.
11. F. Pacini, *Osservazioni microscopiche e deduzioni patologiche sul cholera asiatico [Microscopic Observations and Pathological Deductions on Cholera]*, (Firenze: Bencini, 1854).
12. Cited in Norman Howard-Jones, "Robert Koch and the cholera vibrio: A centenary," *British Medical Journal* 288 (February 4, 1984): pp. 379–81.
13. Ibid.
14. Myron Echenberg, *Africa in the Time of Cholera: A History of Pandemics from 1817 to the Present* (New York, NY: Cambridge University Press, 2011).
15. Ibid., p. 73.
16. Ibid., pp. 76–77.
17. Mariko Ogawa, "Uneasy bedfellows: Science and politics in the refutation of Koch's bacterial theory of cholera," *Bulletin of the History of Medicine* 74 (2000): 671–707; Atalic, "1885 cholera controversy," p. 43.
18. "Further reports by Surgeon-General Hunter on cholera epidemic in Egypt," *Journal of the House of Lords* (C. 4904) (1883), 3–4, cited in Emma Grunberg, "The rationality of inaccurate science: Britain, cholera and the pursuit of progress in 1883," BA Thesis, 2007, Jackson School of International Studies, University of Washington, Seattle, Washington.

Notes—Chapter 12

19. "Cholera in Egypt: The mission of Surgeon-General Hunter: The final report," *The British Medical Journal* 1 (February 9, 1884): 285–87.

20. Ibid.

21. Drs. Timothy Lewis (1841–1886) and David Douglas Cunningham (1843–1914) had previously described amoebic dysentery and leprosy among the population in India. Lewis is also given credit for his discovery of the parasitic worm as the etiological agent of elephantiasis in India in 1872, to which he gave the name *Filaria sanguinis hominis*. His twelve-year career in India included the study of cholera, lending significant credibility to his hypotheses. When Koch later described the comma bacillus he observed in the stools of cholera victims, Lewis' response was "these were nothing more nor less than a *Spirillum* broken by manipulation" (*Nature* 34 [May 27, 1886]: 76–77). Lewis died in 1886, prior to the general acceptance of the cholera bacillus as the agent of the disease. It is suggested he contracted pneumonia by accidentally inoculating himself during his studies.

22. "Cholera in Egypt."

23. John Waller, *The Discovery of the Germ: Twenty Years that Transformed the Way We Think About Disease* (New York, NY: Columbia University Press, 2002).

24. Atalic, "1885 cholera controversy," p. 43.

25. The student of microbiology would be familiar with names of the bacterial genus coined in honor of one of these men: *Nocardia*.

26. Norman Howard-Jones, *The Scientific Background of the International Sanitary Conferences 1851–1938* (Geneva: WHO, 1975), pp. 46–47.

27. Likely rinderpest, a disease cause by a virus similar to that of measles.

28. Howard-Jones, *Scientific Background*, p. 47. A more detailed description is also cited and provided by Gerald Weissmann, ed., "Science in the Middle East: 'Yes, you have found it,'" *The Journal of the Federation of American Societies for Experimental Biology* 20, no. 12 (October 2006): 1943–45. The title of the article, "Yes, you have found it," originates with a myth surrounding Thullier's death. Koch, who was in fact nearby at the time, was alleged to have been present at the bedside when Thullier died. Thullier was said to have asked Koch, "Have we found it?" referring to particles observed in the blood of cholera patients. Koch responded, "Yes, you have found it." Additional information is found in the *Maryland Medical Journal* 10 (November 10, 1883): 458.

29. Howard-Jones, *Scientific Background*, p. 47.

30. Ibid., pp. 47–48.

31. Norman Howard-Jones, "Robert Koch and the cholera vibrio: A centenary," *British Medical Journal* 288 (February 4, 1984): 379–81.

32. Edmund Charles Wendt, ed., *A Treatise on Asiatic Cholera* (New York, NY: William Wood, 1885). Despite the professional courtesy, Cuningham (as he preferred his name to be spelled) remained unconvinced of the contagious nature of the disease. His later response once Koch had announced the discovery of the comma bacillus was the assertion, "The whole superstructure that the German Cholera Commission raised on the supposition that the comma-bacillus is an organism peculiar to cholera, and which was viewed with such ready approval both by the public and a great part of the medical profession has in fact tumbled to the ground." William Guyer Hunter, the British surgeon-general, concurred: "The professional staff, a large body of students and attendants of the Medical College and Hospital, Bombay, who were more or less in frequent communication with cases of cholera ... appeared to enjoy comparative immunity from the disease without any special precautions being taken.... It was no uncommon thing to hear from medical officers and others that their clothing and persons had been covered with the discharges from cholera patients, which had been allowed to become dry, yet no evil results followed" (p. 199).

33. Thomas Brock, *Robert Koch: A Life in Medicine and Bacteriology* (Washington, DC: ASM, 1999).

34. Howard-Jones, *Scientific Background*, p. 49.

35. Ibid.

36. Ibid., p. 50.

37. Ibid.

Notes — Chapter 13

38. Atalic, "1885 cholera controversy," p. 44.
39. Howard-Jones, "Robert Koch," p. 380.
40. Wolfgang Locher, "Max von Pettenkofer — Life stations of a genius on the 100th anniversary of his death (February 9, 1901)," *International Journal of Hygiene and Environmental Health* 203 (2001): 379–91.
41. [Max] von Pettenkofer, Privy Councillor, "On cholera, with reference to the recent epidemic at Hamburg," *The Lancet*, November 19, 1892, 1182–85.
42. Ibid.
43. Locher, "Max von Pettenkofer," p. 384.
44. Pfeiffer is almost forgotten among modern microbiologist, with the exception of being the discoverer of the eponymously named Pfeiffer's bacillus. Also known as *Bacillus influenzae* for its isolation from the lungs of influenza patients, for several decades until the isolation of the actual etiological agent, a virus, the bacterium was thought to be the cause of the disease. Pfeiffer was well known among his contemporaries for his work in immunology.
45. Von Pettenkofer, "On cholera," p. 1182.
46. Even in modern times, skeptics of alleged etiological agents carry out, or at least threaten, to intentionally expose themselves. The author is reminded of Peter Duesberg, a noted retrovirologist who has disputed the role of Human Immunodeficiency Virus (HIV) as the etiological agent of Acquired Immunodeficiency Disease (AIDS). Duesberg has suggested exposing himself in order to test his hypothesis, though to my knowledge he has not done so.
47. Howard-Jones, *Scientific Background*, p. 52.
48. Ibid., p. 53.
49. Ibid., p. 50.
50. Ibid., p. 77.

Chapter 13

1. *The Boston Medical and Surgical Journal* 165, no. 4 (July 27, 1911): 143.
2. Frank Snowden, *Naples in the Time of Cholera, 1884–1911* (New York, NY: Cambridge University Press, 1996).
3. A.E. Newton, K.E. Heiman, A. Schmitz, et al., "Cholera in United States associated with epidemic in Hispaniola," *Emerging Infectious Diseases* 17 (November 2011): 2166–68.
4. Howard Markel, *When Germs Travel: Six Major Epidemics That Have Invaded America and the Fears They Unleashed* (New York: Pantheon, 2004).
5. David Sack et al., "Cholera," *The Lancet* 363 (January 17, 2004): 223–33.
6. F.S. Bunker, "Anti-cholera inoculation," *Science*, November 13, 1885, pp. 439–40. Ferran had based his hypothesis on what had been referred to as the "Depletion Theory," that immunity developed as a result of the depletion of an essential nutrient, either through previous encounter with the agent or as a result of vaccination.
7. Ibid.
8. Ilana Lowy, "From guinea pigs to man: The development of Haffkine's anti-cholera vaccine," *Journal of the History of Medicine and Allied Sciences* 47 (1992): 270–309.
9. Ibid., p. 289.
10. Suman Kanungo and Dipika Sur, "Cholera and its vaccines," *Pediatric Infectious Disease* 4, no. 1 (January–March 2012): 18–24.
11. William van Heyningen and John Seal, *Cholera, The American Scientific Experience, 1947–1980* (Boulder, CO: Westview, 1983), pp. 45–46.
12. Kaushik Bharati and Nirmal Ganguly, "Cholera toxin: A paradigm of a multifunctional protein," *Indian Journal of Medical Research* 133 (February 2011): 179–87.
13. Van Heyningen and Seal, *Cholera*, cited in Robert Hall, "A De in the life of cholera," *Indian Journal of Medical Research* 133 (February 2011): 146–52.
14. S.N. De, "Enterotoxicity of bacteria-free culture filtrate of *Vibrio cholerae*," *Nature* 183 (May 30, 1959): 1533–34.
15. Sack et al., "Cholera;" Nathaniel Pierce, William B. Greenough III, and Charles Carpenter, Jr., "*Vibrio cholerae* enterotoxin and its mode of action," *Bacteriological Reviews* 35, no. 1 (March 1971): 1–13.

Bibliography

Books

Adams, Francis, trans. *The Genuine Works of Hippocrates*. Vol. 1. London: Adlard, 1849.

Algeo, Matthew. *The President Is a Sick Man*. Chicago, IL: Chicago Review Press, 2011.

Ashton, John. "John Snow, the Broad Street Pump and After." In *The Epidemiological Imagination*. Bristol, PA: Open University Press, 1994.

Barnes, Joseph, et al. *The Cholera Epidemic of 1873*. Washington, DC: Government Printing Office, 1875.

Barua, Dhiman, and William B. Greenough III (eds.). *Cholera*. New York: Plenum, 1992.

Bird, Christiane. *The Sultan's Shadow: One Families Rule at the Crossroads of East and West*. New York: Random House, 2010.

Blacker, Valentine. *Memoir of the Operations of the British Army in India During the Mahratta War of 1817–1819*. London: Black, 1821.

Brock, Thomas. *Robert Koch: A Life in Medicine and Bacteriology*. Washington, D.C.: ASM, 1999.

Bunge, William. *Fitzgerald: Geography of a Revolution*. Athens, GA: University of Georgia Press, 2011.

Burton, Clarence Monroe. *Detroit in 1849*. Collection of newspaper accounts, 1910. University of Michigan Library.

Burton, Clarence, ed. *The City of Detroit, Michigan, 1701–1922*. Detroit, MI: S.J. Clarke, 1922.

Campbell, Henry Colin. *Wisconsin in Three Centuries, 1634–1905: Wisconsin as a Territory*. New York: The Publishing Society of New York, 1906.

Chambers, John Sharpe. *The Conquest of Cholera: America's Greatest Scourge*. New York: Macmillan, 1938.

Chardavoyne, David. *A Hanging in Detroit: Stephen Gifford Simmons and the Last Execution Under Michigan Law*. Detroit, MI: Wayne State University Press, 2003.

Daisy, Michael, ed. *Detroit Water and Sewerage Department: The First 300 Years*.

Donald, David Herbert. *Lincoln*. New York: Touchstone, 1996.

Echenberg, Myron. *Africa in the Time of Cholera: A History of Pandemics from 1817 to the Present*. New York: Cambridge University Press, 2011.

Elliott, Charles Winslow. *Winfield Scott: The Soldier and the Man*. New York: Macmillan, 1937.

Farmer, Silas. *History of Detroit and Wayne County*. 3rd ed. Detroit: Silas Farmer, 1890.

Fuller, George Newman. *Economic and Social Beginnings of Michigan*. Lansing, MI: Wynkoop, Hallenbeck Crawford, 1916.

Global Issues in Water, Sanitation and Health: Workshop Summary. Washington, DC: National Academies Press, 2009.

History of Washtenaw County Michigan. Chicago: Charles Chapman, 1881.

Hahnemann, Samuel. *Organon of Medicine*. Blaine, WA: Cooper, 1982.

Bibliography

———. *The Lesser Writings of Samuel Hahnemann.* New York: William Radde, 1852.

Haley, Bruce. *The Healthy Body and Victorian Culture.* Cambridge, MA: Harvard University Press, 1978.

Hemans, Lawton. *Life and Times of Stevens Thomson Mason, the Boy Governor of Michigan.* Lansing, MI: Michigan Historical Commission, 1920.

Heyningen, William van, and John Seal. *Cholera, The American Scientific Experience, 1947–1980.* Boulder, CO: Westview, 1983.

Howard-Jones, Norman. *The Scientific Background of the International Sanitary Conferences 1851–1938.* Geneva: World Health Organization, 1975.

Johnson, Steven. *The Ghost Map.* New York: Penguin, 2006.

Kelly, John. *The Graves Are Walking; The Great Famine and the Saga of the Irish People.* New York: Henry Holt, 2012.

Koeppel, Gerard. *Bond of Union: Building the Erie Canal and the American Empire.* Cambridge, MA: Da Capo, 2009.

Leake, Paul. *A History of Detroit.* Vol. 1. Chicago and New York: Lewis, 1912.

Loomis, Bill. *Detroit's Delectable Past: Two Centuries of Frog Legs, Pigeon Pie and Drugstore Whiskey.* Charleston, SC: History Press, 2012.

Markel, Howard. *When Germs Travel: Six Major Epidemics That Have Invaded America and the Fears They Unleashed.* New York: Pantheon, 2004.

Michigan Pioneer and Historical Society. *Historical Collections.* Lansing, MI: Robert Smith, 1900.

Michigan State Medical Society. *Medical History of Michigan.* Vol. 1. Minneapolis and St. Paul, MN: Bruce, 1903.

Morris, Peter. *Baseball Fever: Early Baseball in Michigan.* Ann Arbor, MI: University of Michigan Press, 2003.

Nevins, Allan, and Milton Halsey Thomas, eds. *The Diary of George Templeton Strong.* Vol. 4. New York: Macmillan, 1952.

Palmer, A.B. *Epidemic Cholera: Its Pathology and Treatment.* Detroit: William Graham, 1866.

Palmer, Friend. *Early Days in Detroit.* Detroit, MI: Hunt and June, 1906.

Parkins, Almon Ernest. *The Historical Geography of Detroit, a Dissertation ... for the Degree of Doctor of Philosophy ... by Almon Ernest Parkins.* Chicago: University Libraries, 1918.

Peeke, Hewson. "The Three Cholera Years." In *A Standard History of Erie County, Ohio.* Chicago and New York: Lewis, 1916.

Quaife, Milo. *Chicago and the Old Northwest: 1673–1835.* Chicago: University of Chicago Press, 2009.

Reynolds, John. *Reynolds' History of Illinois My Own Times : Embracing Also the History of My Life.* Chicago: Chicago Historical Society, 1879.

Roberts, Robert. *Sketches of the City of Detroit.* Detroit: R.F. Johnstone, 1855.

Rosenberg, Charles. *The Cholera Years: The United States in 1832, 1849 and 1866.* Chicago: University of Chicago Press, 1987.

Sengupta, Kaviraj. *The Ayurvedic System of Medicine.* Vol. 2. New Delhi, India: Logos, 1994.

Shattuck, Lemuel. *Report of the Sanitary Commission of Massachusetts 1850.* Boston: Dutton and Wentworth, 1850.

Smith, Arthur. *Old Fuss and Feathers: The Life and Exploits of Lt.-General Winfield Scott.* New York: Greystone, 1937.

Snow, John. *On the Mode of Communication of Cholera.* 2nd ed. London: John Churchill, 1855.

Snowden, Frank. *Naples in the Time of Cholera, 1884–1911.* New York: Cambridge University Press, 1996.

Stein, Mark. *How the States Got Their Shapes.* New York: HarperCollins, 2008.

———. *How the States Got Their Shapes Too: The People Behind the Borderlines.* Washington, DC: Smithsonian Books, 2011.

Bibliography

Stevens, Frank. *The Black Hawk War*. Chicago: Frank E. Stevens, 1903.

13th Annual Report of the Secretary of the State Board of Health of the State of Michigan, for the fiscal year ending September 30, 1885. Lansing, MI: Thorp and Godfrey, 1886.

Waller, John. *The Discovery of the Germ: Twenty Years that Transformed the Way We Think About Disease*. New York: Columbia University Press, 2002.

Weintraub, Stanley. *Victoria: An Intimate Biography*. New York: Dutton Adult/Penguin, 1987.

Welch, Samuel Manning. *Home History: Recollections of Buffalo During the Decade from 1830 to 1840, or Fifty Years Since*. Buffalo: Peter Paul & Bro.,1890.

Wendt, Edmund Charles, ed. *A Treatise on Asiatic Cholera*. New York: William Wood, 1885.

Wentworth, John. *Early Chicago, Fort Dearborn; An Address Delivered at the Unveiling of the Memorial, May 21st, 1881*. Chicago: Fergus, 1881.

Whitney, Ellen, ed. *The Black Hawk War 1831–1832*. Vol. 2, *Letters and Papers*, Part 1. Springfield, IL: Illinois State Historical Library, 1973.

Woodford, Arthur. *This Is Detroit: 1701–2001*. Detroit, MI: Wayne State University Press, 2001.

Woodworth, John, M.D. *Cholera Epidemic of 1873 in the United States*. Washington, DC: Government Printing Office, 1875.

Newspapers and Periodicals

Acta Medica Scandanavica
American Journal of Epidemiology
American Journal of Public Health
American Journal of the Medical Sciences
American Railroad Journal
Association Medical Journal
Bacteriological Reviews
British Journal of Haematology
British Medical Journal
Bulletin of the History of Medicine
Bulletin of the World Health Organization
Christian Inquirer
Cincinnati Commercial
Detroit Daily Free Press
Detroit Review of Medicine and Pharmacy
Emerging Infectious Diseases
Indian Journal of Medical Research
International Journal of Hygiene and Environmental Health
Journal of Chemical Education
Journal of Infectious Diseases
Journal of Medical Ethics
Journal of Public Health Policy
Journal of the History of Medicine and Allied Sciences
Journal of the Michigan State Medical Society
Journal of the Proceedings of the Common Council of the City of Detroit, 1824–1843
Journal of the Royal College of Physicians of Edinburgh
Maryland Medical Journal
Medical and Surgical Reporter
Medical History
Michigan Historical Collections
Michigan History Magazine
Michigan Journal of Homeopathy
Michigan Medicine
Nature
New York Journal
New York Medical Journal
Niles Weekly Register
Old Lead Historical Society
Pediatric Infectious Disease
Peninsular Journal of Medicine and the Collateral Sciences
Pioneer Health
Proceedings of the Royal Society of Medicine
Publications of the Buffalo Historical Society
Science
The American Medical Monthly
The Boston Medical and Surgical Journal
The Buffalonian
The Chicago Tribune
The Democratic Free Press
The Detroit Free Press

Bibliography

The Eclectic Medical Journal
The Journal of the Federation of American Societies for Experimental Biology
The Lancet
The Medical Times and Gazette
The New York Times
Transactions of the Medical Society of the State of New York

Web Sites

http://www.cdc.gov/haiticholera/haiti_cholera.htm

http://www.paho.org/english/sha/epibul_95-98/be971cho.htm

http://classics.mit.edu//Hippocrates/epidemics.html

http://www.globalsecurity.org/wmd/intro/bio_cholera.htm

http://www.ph.ucla.edu/epi/snow/pandemic1826-37.html

http://www.uppercanadahistory.ca/tt/tt1.html

http://www.ncbi.nlm.nih.gov/pmc/articles/PMC233409/pdf/mlab00208-1001.pdf

http://www.collectionscanada.gc.ca/obj/s4/f2/dsk2/ftp01/MQ37236.pdf

http://www.cbc.ca/history/EPISCONTENTSE1EP7CH1PA5LE.html

http://www.bechs.org/exhibits/buffalo_anniversary/175th/page_l1.htm#cholera

http://www.buffalonian.com/history/articles/1801-50/cholera32.html

http://files.usgwarchives.net/mi/downward/multiple/ships/c40002.txt

http://ech.cwru.edu/ech-cgi/article.pl?id=CEO1

http://www.jstor.org/pss/30235761

http://wayne.migenweb.net/boardindex.htm

http://www.illinoisgenealogy.org/rock-island/general_gaines_reply_to_gov_reynolds.htm

http://clarke.cmich.edu/resource_tab/information_and_exhibits/i_arrived_at_detroit/emily_mason.html

http://files.usgwarchives.net/mi/lenawee/history/petition2.txt

https://byustudies.byu.edu/PDFLibrary/44.2RushtonCholera-bb78b7fe-2282-41c9-9ab0-c09b34018536.pdf

http://www.sciencemuseum.org.uk/hommedia.ashx?id=7498&size=Large

http://familytreemaker.genealogy.com/users/s/t/o/Mary-jo-Stoutenburg/PDFGENE6.pdf

http://www.vny.cuny.edu/index-2.html

Index

Abruzzi (steamship) 191
Adams, Capt. John 57
Alexandria, Egypt 182–184
Alger, Gov. Russell 172
Allen, Lewis F. 23, 26
Anderson, Dr. W.J. 136
Atalanta (ship) 146, 151–152, 155
Atkinson, Gen. Henry 56–59

Bailey, Maj. David 56
Batewell (Batwell), Dr. Edward 141
Battle of Bad Axe 58
Battle of Lake Erie 32
Battle of Wisconsin Heights 58
Beaumont, Dr. William 52, 104
Beck, Lewis 21, 22, 28, 29, 30, 200*n*1
Begole, Gov. Josiah 171–172
Belle Isle 43, 203*n*4
Berthelet, Peter 48–49
Black Hawk (Black Sparrow Hawk) (tribal leader) 27, 54–59, 204*n*7
Blackwell, Dr. Elizabeth 109
Boyer, Mrs. Joshua 90
British Commission 180–182, 188–189; *see also* Hunter, William Guyer
Brock, Gen. Sir Isaac 31
Brodie, Dr. William 145–146, 159, 167–168
Brown, Gen. Jacob 36
Brown, Dr. William 104
Browning, Francis 93
Buchanan, Pres. James 202*n*25
Buffalo, New York 3; 1832 epidemic 22–28
Burton, Capt. Josiah 69–71
Burwell, Dr. Bryant 26
Byrd, Dr. J.H. 124, 207*n*17

Cadillac, Antoine de la Mothe 43
Calhoun, Sec. of War John Caldwell 203*n*3
Canada 14, 15, *20*, 21, 48, 65, 111–114, 145, 156, 172, 188; *see also* Lower Canada; Montreal; Quebec City; Upper Canada
Canann, John 96
Canning, Ebenezer 93
Carricks (ship) 15

Cass, Elizabeth 83
Cass, Lewis: as Secretary of War 40, 59, *83*, 83; as territorial governor *48*, 50, 54, 98
Catholic Female Association 95
Centers for Disease Control and Prevention 1, 192
Chadwick, Edwin 175
Champion, Salmon 70
Chapin, Dr. Cyrenius 25
Chapin, Marshall *26*, 53, 66, 90, 204*n*17
Chase, Dr. Alvin Wood 78
Chittenden, Martin 24
Clay, Sen. Henry 62
Clay, Lt. Joseph 36; death 38, 203*n*7
Cobb, Dr. H.P. 106
Cobb, Dr. Lucretius 105
Conger, William 129
Cook, Mayor Levi 66
Council of Hygiene and Public Health 154
Cozens, Isaac 132
Cozens, Sarah 132
Crane, Lt.-Col. Ichabod 28, 201*n*21, 202*n*28
Crittenden, Lt. George 36
Crittenden, Sen. John 36
Crookes, R. William 208*n*9
Cuba 172
Cullen, William 137
Cummings, Lt.-Col. Alexander 40, 201*n*21
Cuningham, Dr. James McNabb 185, 210*n*32
Cunningham, Dr. Douglas 181, 210*n*21

Davis, Lorenzo 69, 73
De, Dr. Sambhu Nath 197
Dequindre, Antoine 83
Dequindre, Catherine 83
Detroit: city health department 51–53, 117, 125–126, 132, 146–148, 160, 164; establishment and development of water and sewage system 47–51, 110–111, 166; founding of city 44–45; War of 1812 30–32, 46
Detroit Medical Society 140
Dodge, Col. Henry 58
Douglass, Silas 130

217

Index

Drummond Island 128
Duesberg, Dr. Peter 211n46
Duffield, Dr. Samuel 126, 148–149

Ege, Dr. Charles 105
Egypt 113, 168–169, 171, 179–180, 184–185, 188–189; *see also* Alexandria; Suez Canal
Elbe (steamship) 175
Ellis, Dr. John 103
England (steamship) 153–154
Erie Canal 23, 46, 200n6
Eustis, Lt.-Col. Abraham 28, 58, 202n28
Everett, Surg. Josiah 37; death 38, 201n21, 203n7
E.W. Stephens (steamboat) 117

Falcon (hospital ship) 152
Farrand, Bethuel 49
Farrand, Dr. David 143–144
Female Medical College 109, 206n12
Ferran y Clua, Dr. Jaime 192–195, 211n6
Fischer, Dr. Bernhard 184
Five Points (area of Manhattan) 120
Florence Nightingale (hospital ship) 152
Florey, Dr. Harold 197
Fort Amherstburg 31, 32
Fort Armstrong 56, 59
Fort Brady 201n22
Fort Columbus 157
Fort Dearborn (Chicago) 36, 38, 41, 43, 58–60, 64, 69
Fort Detroit 31–32
Fort Gratiot **29**, 30–31, 33, 37–38, 40, 43, 47, 62–64, 74, 133, 201n22, 202n33; *see also* Lakeside Cemetery; Port Huron
Fort Jackson 157
Fort Mackinac 27, 41
Fort McHenry 202n26
Fort Shelby 46, **46**; *see also* Fort Detroit
Fox, Reverend Charles 132–133
Franklins (baseball club) 90
French Commission 182–184; *see also* Nocard, Edmond; Roux, Émile; Thuiller, Louis

Gaffky, Dr. George 184, 186, 188
Gaines, Gen. Edmund 55–56
General Lafayette (steamboat) 117
Germ theory of disease 34, 77, 142, 177
German Commission 170, 181, 183–187; *see also* Robert Koch
Goodler, Dr. A.G. 122
Governor's Island 157–158; *see also* Fort Columbus
Gratiot, Charles **28**, 32, 202n33; *see also* Fort Gratiot
Gronasen, Einar 132
Gunn, Dr. Moses 144

Haffkine, Dr. Waldemar 192, 195–196, 211n8
Hahnemann, Dr. Samuel (and homeopathy) 137–140
Haiti 1, 198
Halifax, Nova Scotia 153
Hamtramck, Col. John Frederick 45
Harnold, John 175
Harper, Walter 144
Harper Hospital (establishment of) 144
Harrison, Gen. William Henry 28, 32, 55
Hart's Island 157
Haskins, Roswell 23, 26
Hawthorne, Nathaniel (death of sister) 202n27
Henry, Dr. Stephen 104
Henry Clay (steamboat) 27–28, 30, 36–37, 40, 60–63
Henry IV (ship) 22
Herman Livingston (steamship) 157
Hermani (ship) 152
Heyl, Sergeant Christian (death of) 38, 203n8
Hickok, Nathaniel 79–81
Hirsch, Adam 132
Hitchcock, Capt. Ethan Allen 34
Hippocrates 9, 10
Hoffmann Island 191
Hog Island (Detroit) 37, 40, 43, 61, 79; *see also* Belle Isle
Holmes, Dr. Oliver Wendell, Sr. 143
Houghton, Dr. Douglass 90–91
Hull, William 30, 31, 32
Hunter, Surg.-Gen. William Guyer 180–182, 188, 210n32
Hurd, Dr. Ebenezer 90–91
Hurd, Elizabeth 91
Hurd, Gildersleeve 91
Hyde, Mayor Oliver 128–129

India 2, 4, 9–12, 112, 139, 169, 171, 179–181, 185–186, 188–189
Inglis, Dr. Richard 105
Ireland 14, 15, 16, 111–114, 154
Italy 178, 191

Jackson, Pres. Andrew 27, 54, 57–60
Jenner, Dr. Edward 193, 204n16
Johnson, Dr. Ebenezer 24

Kerr, John 16
Kerr, (Asst.) Surg. Robert 37
Klein, Dr. Peter 105
Knapp, Thomas 93
Koch, Dr. Robert 3, 5, 143, 150; isolation of cholera bacillus 169–170, **171**, 177–179, 181, 183–189, 193, 196–197, 210nn28,32; *see also* Koch's Postulates

218

Index

Koch's Postulates 184–185
Kundig, Father Martin 6, 94, **95**, 95–97

Lagueux, Louis 17
Lakeside Cemetery **31, 32**
Lambeth Company 176
Lane, Marcus 70–73
Larned, Gen. Charles 92
Latta, Dr. Thomas 35, 202n1
Lawton, Dr. A.G. 135
Legionnaire's Disease 5
Le Havre 115–116, 152
Leland, Dr. A.L. 105
Lewis, Dr. Timothy 181, 210n21
Lincoln, Pres. Abraham 54, 57, 204n7
Lind, Dr. James 77
Littré, Paul-Maximillien-Émile 199n2
London Epidemiological Society 181
Lower Canada 3, 19, 23, 200n25

Macomb, Gen. Alexander 36
Macomb, (Asst.) Surg. Edward 201n21
Madison, Pres. James 30–31
Marcus, Rabbi Samuel 132
Marshall, Dr. John 24
Martin, Nancy 144
Mary Ann (ship) 152
Mason, Emily 66
Mason, Gov. Stevens 66, **72**, 73, 75, 91, 96, 99
McCullough, Col. Ben 202n25
McKee, John 16
McKinstry, Col. David 97–98
McMillan, Dr. Robert 90
McNabs Island 153
Metchnikoff, Dr. Elie 195
Michigan State Medical Society 144
La Minerve (newspaper) 16
Moltke (steamship) 191
Montreal 14–17, 19, 20, 28, 44, 48, 114, 172
Mower, Dr. Thomas Gardner 34

New York (packet ship) 115–116, 119
New York City 22, 127; 1866 epidemic 153–156; 1911 outbreak 191–192; *see also* Council of Hygiene and Public Health; Governor's Island; Hart's Island; Swinburne
Noble, Israel 98
Nocard, Dr. Edmond 182–183
Norris, Mark 70
North America (ship) 128
Norton, Walter 36

O'Shaughnessy, Dr. William 35

Pacini, Filippo 4, 178, 189
Palmer, Dr. Alonzo Benjamin 160–163

Paraselsus 123
Pasteur, Dr. Louis 77, 142, 149, **167**, **177**, **181**, 182–183, 193, 204n16
Payne, Maj. Matthew Mountjoy 28, 36, 201n21, 202n26
Peninsular Medical Society 207n3
Perry, Lt. Chester 69
Peruvian (steamship) 154
Pettibone, Samuel 73
Pfeiffer, Dr. Richard 188, 211n44
Phelps, William 76
Phoenix (steamboat) 19
Pierce, Loring 24
Pitcher, Dr. Zina 90, 91, 101, 104, **105**, 106–107, 129–131, 133–134, 141, 143–144, 146–147, 159–160
Polk, Pres. James 117
Port Huron 47, 133, 144, 171
Porter, Gen. Andrew 85
Porter, Dr. Arthur 90
Porter, Dr. David 79
Porter, Gov. David (brother of George) 85
Porter, Gov. George 84–85, **85**, 92
Porter, Sec. of War James Madison 85
Progress (ship) 128

Quebec City 14–17, 19, 20, 28, 114, 200n27

Ransom, Seth 69–70, 73
Reynolds, Gov. John 55–57, 60
Rice, Dr. Randall 51–53, 65, 78, 89–90, 104–105
Richard, Father Gabriel 6, 45, **81**, (death) 82–84
Richardson, Dr. Charles 162
Roux, Dr. Émile **168**, 182
Russell, Dr. George 104
Russia 10, 12

Sac and Fox (tribe) 27, 56–59; *see also* Sauk and Meskwaki
Sampson (steamboat) 116
San Salvador (steamship) 157
Sauk and Meskwaki (tribe) 55
Savannah, Georgia 157, 163; *see also* Tybee Island
Schonbein, Dr. Christian 124
Scott, Gen. Winfield 4, 27–29, 31–32, 34–35, **35**, 36–41, 54, 57–60, 62–64, 69, 201n21, 202n28, 202n2, 203n3
Scovill, Dr. J.B. 90
Selwyn, Sidney 10
Semmelweis, Dr. Ignaz 142–143
Sheldon, John 74, 79
Sheldon Thompson (steamboat) 27, 28, 30, 36, **37**, 38, 40–41, 60, 62–64
Sibley, Judge Solomon 83

219

Index

Silberman, Jacob 132
Simmons, Stephen 93
Skinner, Elias 69
Slayter, Dr. John 153
Smith, Joseph 76
Smith, Asst. Surg. Samuel 66–67
Snow, Dr. John 22, 29, 113, 118, 149, 162, **165**, 174–177, 181, 185–186
Southwark and Vauxhall 176
Spencer, Dr. Silas 90
Sproat, Katherine 83
Stackhouse, Samuel 70–73
Starkey, Henry 90–91; *see also* Franklins
Starkey, Dr. Lewis 90–91, 107
Staten Island 116, 119
Stebbins, Dr. N.B. 90
Stillman, Maj. Isaiah 56–57
Stockwell, Dr. Cyrus 133, 144
Strauss, Dr. Isidore 182
Strong, George Templeton 99
Suez Canal 179, 182
Sumner, Dr. James 209n9
Superior (steamboat) 27, 36, 63
Swartwout, Gen. Robert 36
Swinburne, Dr. John 154
Swinburne Island 191
Sydenham Medical Society 104

Taschereau, Judge Jean Thomas 17
Tecumseh (Shawnee Chief) 31, 92
Temple Beth El 132
Terry, Dr. Adrian 103–104, 106
Thayer, Dr. S.B. Thayer 103
Thompson, Maj. Alexander 64, 201nn21,22
Throop, Gov. Enos 21
Thuiller, Dr. Louis 182–183, 185, 210n28
Tillinghast, Dyre 23
Treaty of Ghent 32, 55
Treaty of Paris 45
Treskow, Dr. Hermann Julius Paul 184
Tripler, Dr. Charles 105
Trowbridge, Mayor Charles 85, *86*
Trowbridge, James 83
Trowbridge, Mary 83
Tuite, Ashleigh 22, 200n4
Turner, Eliphalet 70, 74

Twiggs, Lt.-Col. David Emanuel 28, 36, 37, 40, 62, 202n25
Tybee Island 157
Tyler, Pres. John 85

Union (steamship) 154
United States (schooner) 52, 93
University of Michigan 130, 160
Upper Canada (Ontario) 20, 23

Vache, Dr. Alexander 22, 200n5
Vanderveer, Dr. Adrian 135
Vasseur, Charles 15, 200n27
Virchow, Dr. Rudolph 186
Virginia (steamship) 153–155
Von Bismarck, Chancellor Otto 178, 186
Von Niemeyer, Dr. Felix 150
Von Pettenkofer, Dr. Max 5, 149–151, 162, *172*, 187–188
Voyageur (ship) 15, 16

Walker, Augustus 62
War of 1812 25, 27, 34, 46, 55, 57, 83, 85, 92, 202nn26,28
Ward's Island 152
Warrior (steamer) 59
Wayne County Medical Society (founded) 105, 143–145, 166; *see also* Michigan State Medical Society
Welch, Samuel 24
Wells, Rufus 49
Westervelt, Dr. John 22
White, Henry 24
Whiting, Dr. John Leffingwell 51–53, 65, 90
Wight, Dr. Orlando Williams 168–170, 172
William Penn (steamboat) 27, 36, 63
Windsor, Ontario 31, 60
Witherell, Benjamin 94
Witherell, Mary 94
Woodward, Judge Augustus 45
World Health Organization 193
Worth, Col. William Jenkins 28, **39**; death 117, 202n28

Ypsilanti, Michigan 68–73

www.ingramcontent.com/pod-product-compliance
Ingram Content Group UK Ltd.
Pitfield, Milton Keynes, MK11 3LW, UK
UKHW041952140426
5217IPUK00015B/769